Get Through

FRCA Physics: MCQs

D1427319

Get Through
FRCA Physics: MCQs

Raja LA Jayaweera MA LLB MBBS DA FRCA
Formerly Consultant Anaesthetist, Whittington Hospital, London

Ramanie Jayaweera MBBS FRCA
Provisional Fellow in Paediatric Anaesthesia, Children's Hospital, Westmead,
Sydney, Australia

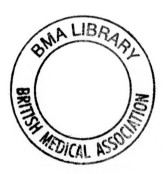

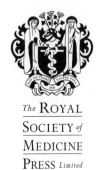

The ROYAL
SOCIETY *of*
MEDICINE
PRESS *Limited*

© 2007 Royal Society of Medicine Press Ltd

Published by the Royal Society of Medicine Press Ltd
1 Wimpole Street, London W1G 0AE, UK
Tel: +44 (0)20 7290 2921
Fax: +44 (0)20 7290 2929
E-mail: publishing@rsm.ac.uk
Website: www.rsmpress.co.uk

British Library Cataloguing in Publication Data
A catalogue record for this book is available from the British Library

ISBN 1-85315-689-2

Distribution in Europe and Rest of World:

Marston Book Services Ltd
PO Box 269
Abingdon
Oxon OX14 4YN, UK
Tel: +44 (0)1235 465500
Fax: +44 (0)1235 465555
Email: direct.order@marston.co.uk

Distribution in the USA and Canada:

Royal Society of Medicine Press Ltd
c/o BookMasters, Inc.
30 Amberwood Parkway
Ashland, Ohio 44805, USA
Tel: +1 800 247 6553/ +1 800 266 5564
Fax: +1 419 281 6883
Email: order@bookmasters.com

Distribution in Australia and New Zealand:

Elsevier Australia
30–52 Smidmore Street
Marrikville NSW 2204, Australia
Tel: +61 2 9349 5811
Fax: +61 2 9349 5911
Email: service@elsevier.com.au

Typeset by Phoenix Photosetting, Chatham, Kent, UK
Printed and bound by Bell & Bain Ltd, Glasgow, UK

Contents

Preface   vii
Abbreviations   ix
Recommended reading   x

Section 1
Text Book: Questions   1
Text Book: Answers   56

Section 2
Practice Paper 1: Questions   127
Practice Paper 1: Answers   137

Practice Paper 2: Questions   151
Practice Paper 2: Answers   160

Practice Paper 3: Questions   171
Practice Paper 3: Answers   180

Practice Paper 4: Questions   191
Practice Paper 4: Answers   200

Practice Paper 5: Questions   213
Practice Paper 5: Answers   223

Appendix 1: Isomerism   237
Appendix 2: SI units   241

Preface

While there are several British textbooks on the physics of anaesthesia there appears to be a dearth of teaching aids on the subject in the form of MCQs for the FRCA examinations. The authors make no claims that the questions here comprehensively cover the subject of anaesthetic physics, yet hope that this book will go some way to fill the need of junior anaesthetist examinees.

Although, for reasons of brevity, it is titled 'FRCA Physics', the book includes questions on some aspects of anaesthetic chemistry, in particular isomerism, as well as on anaesthetic equipment, with the occasional foray into those aspects of physiology and pharmacology that have a 'physical' basis.

Inevitably, where a large number of MCQs needs to be provided there is bound to be some repetition of subject matter, and in that respect this book is no different from most MCQs books. Arguably, such repetition could be regarded as desirable for it may aid the learner by providing opportunity for recapitulation and therefore revision.

The book is arranged in two parts: 'Text Book', which contains 304 questions, arranged according to subject matter, followed by five 'Practice Papers', each containing 50 questions. Answers and explanations are provided for each of the sections.

In addition, there are two 'appendices', one on SI units and the other on isomerism, neither of which subjects appears to be adequately covered in conventional anaesthetic textbooks.

This book is intended for those preparing for the Primary FRCA examination, but it could be equally useful as a revision aid for the Final Fellowship.

Raja LA Jayaweera
Ramanie Jayaweera

Abbreviations

AP	anaesthetic-proof
APG	anaesthetic-proof gas
APL	adjustable pressure limiting
BP	blood pressure
CFC	chlorofluorocarbon
cgs	centimetre gram second
CNS	central nervous system
CVP	central venous pressure
DBS	double-burst stimulation
EMF	electromotive force
EMR	electromagnetic radiation
ERG	electroretinogram
FCG	French catheter gauge
IPPV	intermittent positive pressure ventilation
LCD	liquid crystal display
MAC	minimum alveolar concentration
MRI	magnetic resonance imaging
PNS	peripheral nerve stimulator
REM	return electrode monitoring
RMS	root mean square
SELV	safety extra low voltage
SVP	saturated vapour pressure
SWG	steel wire guage
TENS	transcutaneous electrical nerve stimulation
TOF	Train-of-Four
TUR	transurethral resection
VF	ventricular fibrillation
VIE	vacuum-insulated evaporator

Recommended reading

Kenny G, Davis P D. Basic Physics and Measurement in Anaesthesia, 5th edn. Oxford: Butterworth-Heinemann, 2003.

Magee P, Tooley M. The Physics, Clinical Measurement and Equipment of Anaesthetic Practice. Oxford: Oxford University Press, 2005.

Moyle J T B, Davey A. Ward's Anaesthetic Equipment, 5th edn. London: WB Saunders, 2006.

Sykes M K, Vickers M D, Hull C J. Principles of measurement and monitoring in anaesthesia and intensive care, 3rd edn. Blackwell Science, Oxford, 1991.

Text book

Quantities, units and basic mathematics

1   The SI convention of units:

   a. Was formally introduced in about 1950.
   b. Is a 'gravitational system' of units.
   c. Is a metric system.
   d. Is based on the cgs (centimetre gram second) system.
   e. Incorporates the angstrom as one of its units of length.

2   In the Système International d'Unités:

   a. There are nine base quantities.
   b. All the quantities are 'extensive', i.e. they all possess additional fiduciary marks.
   c. The unit of *length* (metre) is now defined by reference to the wavelengths of the krypton nuclide.
   d. *Luminance* is one of the base quantities.
   e. The unit of *Quantity of Substance* (mole) is defined by reference to hydrogen.

3   In the conventions for writing SI units:

   a. The names of units when written in full shall commence with an upper case letter.
   b. Abbreviation symbols shall employ an upper case first letter whenever the unit is named after a person.
   c. The abbreviations shall have no plural form.
   d. Punctuation marks shall be used with abbreviations, e.g. '1 kg.' (i.e. a *dot* after 'kg').
   e. The abbreviation for 'metre' is 'M' (i.e. an upper case M).

4   The following statements are correct with respect to the SI units system:

   a. The abbreviation for 'decibel' is 'Db'.
   b. 'Kilopascals' is denoted by the abbreviation 'Kpa'.
   c. The 'litre' is an SI unit of volume.
   d. A temperature of 273 kelvin is correctly abbreviated to '273 °Kelvin'.
   e. The letter 'G' stands for 'gray', the absorbed dose of radiation.

5   The following abbreviations are correct:

   a. Cu for curie, the non-SI unit of radioactivity.
   b. B for Becquerel, the SI unit of radioactivity.
   c. Z for atomic number.
   d. R for electrical impedance.
   e. S for sievert, the SI unit of dose equivalent in radiation.

1

6   The following quantities are correctly denoted in accordance with the SI convention for writing units:

a. A frequency of 25 Hertz as '25 hz'. F
b. A length of 100 000 centimetres as '10^5 cm'. F
c. One litre as '10^3 cc'. F
d. 1 atmosphere pressure as '10^5 pascals'. F
e. A speed of 100 kilometres per second as '100 km/s'. F

7   The following are base units in the SI units system:

a. Metre. T
b. Radian. F
c. Lumen. F
d. Coulomb. F
e. Farad. F

8   The following are regarded as 'supplementary' units under the SI nomenclature:

a. Radian. T
b. Electron-volt. F
c. Ångstrom. F
d. Centimetres water (as a unit of pressure). F
e. Steradian. T

9   The following are non-SI units:

a. Kilopascal. F
b. Ångstrom. T
c. Joule. F
d. Electron-volt. T
e. Millimetre mercury. T

10   The following are SI units:

a. Dyne. F
b. Stokes. F
c. Henry. T
d. Poise. F
e. Siemens. T

11   The following are SI units:

a. Farad.
b. Talbot.
c. Tesla.
d. Becquerel.
e. Gray.

12   The following are base units under the SI system:

a. Calorie. F
b. Candela. T
c. Celsius. T
d. Centimetre. F
e. Coulomb. F

13 In the SI units system the metre has been correctly defined as follows:

 a. One ten millionth part of the earth's meridian quadrant (distance from the North Pole to the Equator) passing through Paris. *F*
 b. The length of a platinum iridium bar of standard length in Sèvres, Paris. *T*
 c. One-thousandth of a kilometre. *F*
 d. Number of wavelengths in a vacuum of the radiations corresponding to transitions in the nuclide krypton-86. *T*
 e. By reference to the speed of light in air. *F*

14 One mole:

 a. Is a base quantity in the SI units system. *T*
 b. Is that amount of substance that contains as many elementary particles as there are atoms in 0.012 kg of carbon-12.
 c. Has 6.02×10^{26} elementary particles in it. *F*
 d. Will always exert an osmolarity of 1 osmol L^{-1} of solution.
 e. Is a necessary entity in determining the value of the ideal gas constant. *F*

15 In the system of units of pressure:

 a. 1 atmosphere is equivalent to approximately 101.325 newtons per square metre.
 b. The torr differs from the mmHg by less than 1/1000.
 c. The actual pressure is always greater than the gauge pressure by 1 standard atmosphere. *F*
 d. 1 newton per square metre pressure is of lesser magnitude than 1 mmHg. *T*
 e. 1 centimetre water pressure is equivalent to 10.0 pascals. *F*

16 The following are approximate equivalents of 1 atmosphere pressure:

 a. 0.76 metres of mercury. *T*
 b. 10 metres water. *F*
 c. 100 000 dynes cm^{-2}. *F*
 d. 1000 kilopascals. *F*
 e. 14 pounds per square inch. *T*

17 The following are correct definitions of the joule:

 a. The work done when a charge of 1 coulomb is moved through a potential difference of 1 volt.
 b. The work done when a current of 1 ampere flows through a resistance of 1 ohm in 1 second.
 c. The energy produced when a power of 1 watt is dissipated in 1 second.
 d. The work done when a force of 1 newton acts through a distance of 1 metre.
 e. The heat required to raise the temperature of 1 gram of water through 1 °C.

18   The unit of 'newtons per metre' is:

a. The conventional mode of expressing surface tension.
b. An essential factor in the SI definition of the ampere.
c. The mode of expressing electromagnetic field strength.
d. The unit of pressure.
e. The unit of 'shear stress' in a flowing fluid.

19   The dimensions of newtons per square metre correctly express:

a. Pressure.
b. Stress.
c. Strain.
d. Surface tension.
e. Gravitational field strength.

20   The following are exact or near-exact equivalents of each other:

a. 1 metre and 1000 millimetres.
b. 1 litre and one-thousandth of a cubic metre.
c. 1 °C and 1 kelvin.
d. 1 torr and 1 mmHg pressure.
e. 1000 newtons per square metre and 1 kilopascal.

21   The following equations are correct:

a. Joule = newton metres.
b. Volt = watts per ampere.
c. Henry = webers per ampere.
d. Farad = coulombs per volt.
e. Watts = joule seconds.

22   The graduations on the following measuring devices are linear (i.e. they are equidistant):

a. Mercury sphygmomanometer.
b. Mercury clinical thermometer.
c. Bourdon pressure gauge on an oxygen cylinder.
d. Nitrous oxide flowmeter tube on an anaesthetic machine.
e. Wright respirometer.

23   The following refer to the same thing:

a. Resonant frequency and natural frequency.
b. Dielectric constant and relative permittivity.
c. Natural logarithms and Briggsian logarithms.
d. Critical damping and optimal damping.
e. Fluid flow rate and fluid flow velocity.

24   The following are correct units for expressing surface tension:

a. Newtons per metre.
b. Dynes per decimetre.
c. Joules per square metre.
d. Watt-seconds per square centimetre.
e. Kilograms per square metre per second.

25 **In the case of an exponential process:**

a. Its behaviour is the same as that of a zero-order process.
b. The rate of change of its variable is proportional to the magnitude of the variable.
c. It can mathematically never come to an end.
d. It nears completion in 3 time constants.
e. In the case of decay of a radioisotope its half-life is greater than its time constant.

26 **The following physical phenomena are exponential in nature:**

a. Radioactive decay.
b. Attenuation of the energy of electromagnetic radiations with distance during transmission through matter.
c. Reduction of the volume of a fixed mass of gas, at constant pressure, in relation to decrease in temperature.
d. Saturation vapour pressure of water and environmental temperature.
e. Solubility of a gas in a liquid and the partial pressure of the gas in the liquid.

27 **The following are parabolic:**

a. Trajectory of an electron in a uniform electrical field.
b. Graphic relationship between pressure and volume in accordance with Boyle's Law.
c. Graph of relationship between frequency of AC electricity and the threshold current that causes ventricular fibrillation.
d. Velocity profile of a fluid front in laminar flow.
e. Magnetization–demagnetization curve for a ferromagnetic material.

28 **The phenomenon of hysteresis is demonstrated by the following:**

a. Intra-alveolar pressure change in the inspiratory and expiratory phases of spontaneous ventilation.
b. Variation with temperature of the pressure of a fixed mass of gas at constant volume.
c. Temperature change when measured with a thermistor during a heating and cooling cycle.
d. Measurement of temperature change by use of colour-sensitive liquid crystal display devices.
e. Magnetization–demagnetization curve for a ferromagnetic material.

29 **The inverse square law correctly applies to the following:**

a. Variation of intensity of a laser light beam with distance of propagation.
b. Magnitude of the product of mutual forces between two electrostatic charges and the distance between them.
c. Rate of diffusion of a substance down its concentration gradient and the molecular weight of the substance.
d. Amplitude of EMR waves and their energy content.
e. Electrical resistance of a conductor and its cross-sectional area.

30   The following when graphically displayed take the form of a rectangular hyperbola:

a. Relationship between volume and pressure of a fixed mass of gas in accordance with Boyle's Law.
b. Substrate concentration and V_0 (initial rate of reaction) in relation to Michaelis–Menten kinetics of enzyme action.
c. Oxygen saturation of myoglobin and the partial pressure of oxygen.
d. Stimulus strength and stimulus duration required for depolarization of a nerve or muscle membrane.
e. Log dose–response curve for a pharmacological agonist.

31   The phenomenon of hysteresis is shown by the following:

a. Stretching and compression cycles of rubber.
b. Intrapleural pressure change during IPPV with a constant pressure generator ventilator.
c. Intra-alveolar pressure change during IPPV with a constant flow generator ventilator.
d. Temperature change of a thermostat controlling a source of heat.
e. Liquid–solid phase transitions for water.

32   The following have an 'A is proportional to B^2' relationship:

a. The amplitude of EMR waves and the energy of the waves.
b. The pressure differential and the flow rate in turbulent flow.
c. Flow rate in laminar flow and cross-sectional area of conduit.
d. Energy of electromagnetic radiations and their Kelvin temperature.
e. Frequency of ultrasound waves and their degree of absorption by the medium of transmission.

33   The following have a direct relationship:

a. Angular frequency ω (in radians per second) of precessing protons (during MRI) and the static magnetic field B_o (in tesla).
b. Michaelis constant (K_m) and enzyme affinity for a substrate.
c. Solubility of a gas in a liquid and the temperature of the liquid.
d. Diamagnetic property of a material and its Kelvin temperature.
e. Frequency of ultrasound waves and their degree of resolution.

34   The following have a direct linear relationship:

a. Partial pressure of a gas in a liquid and the amount of the gas in simple solution in the liquid.
b. Viscosity of blood and its haematocrit.
c. Pressure of oxygen inside an oxygen cylinder and the amount of oxygen inside the cylinder.
d. Amount of water vapour in the atmosphere and the atmospheric pressure.
e. Frequency of ultrasound waves and their degree of penetration.

35   **The following when graphically represented take the form of an accelerating growth exponential:**

a. Haematocrit and blood viscosity.
b. Saturation vapour pressure of a liquid and its ambient temperature.
c. Conductivity of a semiconductor in relation to its temperature.
d. Velocity of flow and viscosity of a thixotropic fluid (such as blood).
e. Inspiratory flow rate during IPPV with a constant pressure generator ventilator.

36   **The following when graphically displayed have a sigmoid configuration:**

a. Haemoglobin–oxygen dissociation curve and partial pressure of oxygen.
b. Michaelis–Menten curve: relationship between the concentration of a substrate and the rate of the corresponding enzyme-controlled reaction.
c. Agonist concentration–receptor occupancy curve for a drug.
d. Thermo-electric EMF as a function of temperature in the case of a thermocouple.
e. Intensity of magnetization of a ferromagnet in relation to the magnetic flux density of the magnetizing field.

37   **The following phenomena exhibit time-related variation of a sinusoidal nature:**

a. RMS voltage of mains electricity.
b. Voltage of an isolated diathermy (electrosurgical) unit.
c. Amplitude of the energy wave of laser light.
d. Energy discharge from an activated DC defibrillator.
e. Amplitude of vibrations of a fluid-coupled transducer for invasive arterial BP monitoring.

38   **The following are temperature dependent:**

a. Radioactive decay.
b. Speed of light in a vacuum.
c. Osmolality.
d. Viscosity of a liquid.
e. Latent heat of vaporization of a halogenated inhalational anaesthetic agent.

39   **The following vary with ambient pressure:**

a. Boiling point of a liquid.
b. Saturation vapour pressure of a liquid inhalational anaesthetic agent.
c. Rate of decay of a radionuclide.
d. Viscosity of a gas.
e. Latent heat of vaporization of water.

40   The following are units of 'rating', i.e. each of them expresses the occurrence of a phenomenon in relation to unit time:

a. Ampere.
b. Watt.
c. Lux.
d. Tesla.
e. Becquerel.

41   The following are 'intensity' units, i.e. they express the occurrence of a phenomenon in relation to unit surface area:

a. Weber.
b. Lux.
c. Lumen.
d. Ampere.
e. Pascal.

42   The following are 'dimensionless entities':

a. Atomic number.
b. Relative atomic mass.
c. Atomic mass number.
d. Atomic mass unit.
e. Atomic weight.

43   The following are 'dimensionless entities':

a. Stress.
b. Strain.
c. Permeability (of a membrane).
d. Partition coefficient.
e. Substitution index.

44   The following are 'dimensionless entities':

a. Hüfner constant.
b. Michaelis constant.
c. Faraday constant.
d. Stefan constant.
e. Avogadro's constant.

45   The following are 'dimensionless entities':

a. Dibucaine number.
b. Reynolds number.
c. Coordination number.
d. Loschmidt's number.
e. Avogadro's number.

46   The following are 'dimensionless entities':

a. Acoustic impedance.
b. Diffusion constant.
c. Specific gravity.
d. Dielectric constant.
e. Universal gas constant.

47   The following are 'dimensionless entities':

   a. Fluoride number.
   b. Quetelet index.
   c. Van't Hoff factor.
   d. Damping coefficient.
   e. Gyromagnetic ratio.

48   The following are 'dimensionless entities':

   a. Dalton.
   b. Normality of a solution.
   c. Permeability of free space
   d. Permittivity of free space.
   e. Mole.

49   The following have the same units:

   a. Pressure and stress.
   b. Luminance and illuminance.
   c. Dynamic viscosity and kinematic viscosity.
   d. Electrical resistance and electrical reactance.
   e. Work and heat quantity.

50   Each of the following pairs of units denotes the same physical
      quantity or phenomenon:

   a. Stokes and poise.
   b. Curie and becquerel.
   c. Henry and weber.
   d. Gauss and tesla.
   e. Coulomb and joule.

51   Each of the following pairs of units denotes the same physical
      quantity or phenomenon:

   a. Rad and gray.
   b. Siemens and mho.
   c. Dyne and newton.
   d. Torr and pascal.
   e. Sievert and rem.

52   Each of the following pairs of units denotes the same physical
      quantity or phenomenon:

   a. Weber and maxwell.
   b. Electron-volt and volt.
   c. Erg and joule.
   d. Lumen and talbot.
   e. Dalton and atomic mass unit.

53   The conditions under which the inverse square law can correctly apply to light include the following:

a. The source of light must be a 'point' source.
b. The source must be 'isotropic'.
c. There must be no absorption or scattering of the radiant energy.
d. There must be no back-scattering of the radiant energy from objects beyond the point of measurement.
e. The radiant light beam must possess the attribute of collimation.

54   The following are examples of transducers:

a. Thermistor probe.
b. A light-emitting diode.
c. A piezo-electric crystal in an ultrasound scanner.
d. The transformer at an electrical substation.
e. The phosphor in an electric fluorescent light tube.

55   Kinetic energy:

a. Is dependent on the velocity of the body to which it refers.
b. Is independent of the body's mass.
c. Is correctly measurable in joules.
d. Is decreased at the point of constriction in a conduit in which fluid flows.
e. Increases progressively in the case of an object when it is thrown up in the air.

56   The following statements are true:

a. All materials are diamagnetic in nature.
b. All bodies emit electromagnetic radiations.
c. All gases necessarily become solids at near 0 kelvin.
d. All biochemically active amino acids in the body are α amino acids.
e. All food carbohydrates are absorbed in the gut as monosaccharides.

57   The following have values in the range of kilohertz and not megahertz:

a. 'Interrogation current' of an REM (return electrode monitoring) diathermy plate.
b. 'Harmonic scalpel' (ultrasound diathermy unit).
c. Operational frequency of the microwave oven.
d. EMR frequency of the CO_2 laser.
e. Long wave radiofrequency waves.

Behaviour of gases and liquids

58   The viscosity of a liquid:

   a. Varies directly with its temperature.
   b. Bears a direct relationship to its specific density.
   c. Is a factor in determining its laminar flow.
   b. Is a factor in determining its Reynolds number.
   e. Is correctly expressed in the units of 'pascals per second'.

59   The density of a fluid is a material factor in the following situations:

   a. In laminar flow in a tube.
   b. In determining the kinematic viscosity of the fluid.
   c. During low gas flows along the tubes of the flowmeter unit of an anaesthetic machine.
   d. In determining the heat capacity of a mass of metal.
   e. In the ease of air flow at the glottis.

60   Both density *and* viscosity play a part in the following:

   a. Flow of gases up an anaesthetic machine flowmeter tube.
   b. Quantification of the flow rate in laminar flow.
   c. Computation of the Reynolds number.
   d. Determination of the kinematic viscosity of a gas.
   e. Use of heliox in the management of laryngeal obstruction.

61   The following are definitional attributes of an 'ideal gas':

   a. It consists of 'dimensionless entities'.
   b. The interparticle forces of attraction in it are negligible.
   c. The collisions of the particles with the container bounding walls are perfectly elastic.
   d. Van der Waals interactions are a standard attribute.
   e. It has a critical temperature below 0 °C.

62   In the case of an 'ideal gas':

   a. Its behaviour is in accordance with van der Waals equation of state.
   b. Its internal energy is entirely kinetic.
   c. Its internal energy is dependent only on temperature.
   d. Its latent heat of vaporization is the same at all temperatures.
   e. It will remain gaseous even at a temperature of near 0 kelvin.

63   Each of the following laws or equations is pertinent in respect of the phenomenon or situation it refers to:

a. Ideal gas equation in determining the amount of oxygen remaining in a cylinder.
b. Charles' Law in determining the internal volume of an air cylinder.
c. Hagen–Poiseuille equation in determining the relationship between shear rate and shear stress of a fluid conforming to turbulent flow.
d. Gay-Lussac's Law in the provision of a supersaturated vapour by the TEC 6 desflurane vaporizer.
e. Boyle's Law in respect of the operation of an autoclave.

64   Raoult's Law:

a. Only applies to ideal solutions.
b. In general only holds for dilute solutions.
c. Is applicable to perfect solutions.
d. Does not hold for azeotropes.
e. Is obeyed by volatile anaesthetic agents in respect of their solubility over clinical ranges of concentrations.

65   The physical principle enshrined in Gay-Lussac's Law ('law of pressures') is an operational principle in the following devices:

a. Vaporization of the agent in the desflurane Mark 6 vaporizer.
b. Provision of superheated steam for sterilization in an autoclave.
c. Use of the Bourdon gauge principle in measuring temperature change in a system.
d. Air entrainment in the performance of a 'fixed performance' oxygen mask.
e. Use of a Pitot tube to measure flow.

66   At its critical temperature:

a. A gas has the same density as its liquid.
b. A gas has a latent heat of vaporization of 0.
c. A gas most closely conforms to an 'ideal gas'.
d. A gas can be liquefied by pressure alone.
e. A gas exhibits no van der Waals forces between its molecules.

67   A Newtonian fluid can be said to have the following:

a. A parabolic profile for its fluid flow front.
b. A flow rate proportional to the square root of the pressure gradient.
c. A viscosity dependent on its flow rate.
d. A flow rate inversely proportional to the specific density of the fluid.
e. A flow rate proportional to the square of the cross-sectional area of the conduit.

68   The vapour pressure of an inhalational anaesthetic agent is
      dependent on:

      a. Atmospheric pressure.
      b. Ambient temperature.
      c. Boiling point of the agent.
      d. Molecular weight of the agent.
      e. Viscosity of the liquid agent.

69   Water:

      a. Is a polar compound.
      b. Is a linear molecule.
      c. Has a high dielectric constant.
      d. When mixed with polar molecules weakens the interactions
         between the latter.
      e. Absorbs UV light.

70   Water:

      a. Has a permanent dipole moment.
      b. Is an amphiphilic compound.
      c. Strongly absorbs EMRs in the infrared region.
      d. Is a good solvent for aromatic compounds.
      e. Is strongly hydrogen bonded.

71   The following are Newtonian or near-Newtonian fluids:

      a. Water.
      b. Saline.
      c. Plasma.
      d. Normal whole blood.
      e. Washed red cells suspended in saline.

Temperature measurement

72   The thermodynamic scale of temperature:

      a. Is an absolute scale of temperature.
      b. Is the same as the kelvin scale.
      c. Is identical to the scale based on the variation of pressure with
         temperature of a fixed mass of an ideal gas at constant volume.
      d. Is independent of the properties of any particular substance.
      e. Has a unit identical in magnitude to that of the celsius scale.

73   The following increase with a rise in temperature:

      a. The solubility of a gas in a liquid.
      b. The rate of disintegration of a radionuclide.
      c. The partial pressure of the vapour of a liquid anaesthetic agent.
      d. The viscosity of a liquid.
      e. The speed of light in a vacuum.

74 The following are temperature dependent:

   a. Electrical conductivity of a semiconductor.
   b. Osmolality of a nonpolar solution.
   c. Ferromagnetic property of a metal.
   d. Diamagnetic property of a gas.
   e. Frequency of EMRs emitted by a body.

75 Temperature measurement can be effected by:

   a. A dimensional change in matter.
   b. A frequency change of EMRs (electromagnetic radiations).
   c. A resistance change in an electrical circuit.
   d. A pressure change in a gas system.
   e. A voltage change in a transistor.

76 The following thermometers have a positive temperature coefficient:

   a. Mercury clinical thermometer.
   b. Gas thermometer.
   c. Platinum resistance thermometer.
   d. Thermocouple.
   e. Thermistor.

77 The following thermometers show a linear change with temperature over their range of operation:

   a. Platinum resistance thermometer.
   b. Thermistor.
   c. Thermocouple.
   d. Mercury clinical thermometer.
   e. Gas thermometer.

78 The following are relevant to the workings of the infrared thermometer:

   a. Wien's Law of displacement.
   b. Stefan–Boltzmann equation.
   c. Planck constant.
   d. Larmor frequency.
   e. Soret peak.

79 The following are potential disadvantages of thermistors as temperature measuring devices:

   a. 'Ageing', i.e. showing resistance change with time.
   b. Tendency to exhibit hysteresis.
   c. Low temperature coefficients of resistance.
   d. Slow response time.
   e. Nonlinearity of resistance change with temperature.

80 The following thermometers determine temperature by detecting a change in electrical resistance in the measuring device:

a. Platinum resistance thermometer.
b. Thermistor.
c. Thermocouple.
d. Bimetallic strip.
e. Bourdon gauge thermometer.

81 In the case of the mercury clinical thermometer:

a. It is a transducer.
b. It determines temperature change by effecting a dimensional change in matter.
c. It uses mercury because mercury has a high coefficient of expansion.
d. It incorporates a lens for rendering the reading of the temperature easier.
e. It now should not be used because of EC regulations.

82 The platinum resistance thermometer:

a. Has a high temperature coefficient of resistance.
b. Has a wide measurement range.
c. Has a relatively large heat capacity.
d. Is more sensitive than the thermistor.
e. Has a faster response time than the thermistor.

83 The thermistor has the following advantages over the platinum resistance thermometer:

a. It is more robust.
b. It is more stable.
c. It is more sensitive.
d. It has a smaller thermal capacity.
e. It has a faster response time.

Anaesthetic gases

84 The amount of the agent contained in each of the following cylinders can be determined by application of the Universal Gas equation:

a. Oxygen cylinder.
b. Nitrous oxide cylinder.
c. Helium/oxygen (79%/21%) cylinder.
d. Air cylinder.
e. Cyclopropane cylinder.

85   Carbon dioxide:

a. Is fully oxidized carbon and cannot therefore be further oxidized.
b. Is produced for medical use by fractional distillation of air.
c. Is formed during anaerobic metabolism.
d. Causes collision broadening during measurement of N_2O by infrared analysis.
e. When reacting with soda lime does so as an endothermic reaction.

86   Carbon dioxide:

a. Is more potent than CFCs (chlorofluorocarbons) as a greenhouse gas.
b. Has a higher critical temperature than nitrous oxide.
c. Has a greater affinity for haemoglobin than carbon monoxide.
d. Has a greater viscosity than oxygen.
e. Is found in a greater percentage in air than is helium.

87   The following relate to the in vivo behaviour of oxygen:

a. Pasteur point.
b. Hüfner constant.
c. Peltier effect.
d. Hamburger phenomenon.
e. Circe effect.

88   Oxygen:

a. Is a paramagnetic gas.
b. Is a diradical.
c. Has an indefinite half-life in nature.
d. Is a prescription-only medicine.
e. Can be analysed by mass spectrometry.

89   Oxygen:

a. Is normally present in a greater volume in the body than is nitrogen.
b. In its gaseous form has a higher viscosity than nitrous oxide.
c. Has a constant percentage in atmospheric air no matter at what height above sea level.
d. Is present in nature as three allotropes.
e. Exists in nature in three stable isotopic forms.

90   Oxygen:

a. Is a polar substance.
b. Exists in radioactive isotope form in nature.
c. Has a critical pressure of about 5000 kPa.
d. Is absorbed by infrared radiation in the atmosphere.
e. Is converted by ultraviolet light to ozone.

91   The manufacture of oxygen can involve the following:

    a. Joule–Thomson effect.
    b. Allis–Chalmers process.
    c. Poynting effect.
    d. Hampson–von Linde process.
    e. Paul Bert effect.

92   Oxygen can be analysed by the following methods:

    a. Mass spectrometry.
    b. Raman scattering.
    c. Polarography.
    d. Infrared analysis.
    e. Paramagnetic analysis.

93   If breathed under hyperbaric conditions, oxygen can give rise to the following:

    a. Paul Bert effect.
    b. Cushing effect.
    c. Lorrain–Smith effect.
    d. Poseiro effect.
    e. Fahraeus–Lindqvist effect.

94   Oxygen:

    a. May be inhaled indefinitely at an FiO_2 of 0.5 at atmospheric pressure without any permanent damage.
    b. If inhaled at 100% under normobaric conditions for 2 hours can cause tightness of the chest.
    c. If breathed at an FiO_2 of 1.0 at 3 atmospheres pressure can cause neurological damage.
    d. If breathed pure is known to decrease velocity of movement of tracheal mucus.
    e. Has been known to cause death from pulmonary oedema.

95   In the case of an oxygen cylinder:

    a. When full, it has a gauge pressure of about 137 bar, no matter the size of cylinder.
    b. Its pressure may be correctly regarded as a manifestation of kinetic energy.
    c. Its gauge pressure is an accurate indicator of the amount of oxygen present in the cylinder.
    d. It suffers the 'Poynting effect' on being exposed to cold temperatures.
    e. It has a higher filling ratio for the tropics than for temperate climates.

96　The following are mandatory rules in respect of the construction and siting of a VIE (vacuum insulated evaporator) supply of oxygen:

a. It shall be in the open air.
b. It shall have no overhead electrical wires or cables.
c. There shall be no ditches or trenches in its vicinity.
d. It shall have no other sources of medical gases adjacent to it.
e. It shall have a pressure relief valve operational at about 700 kPa.

97　Ozone:

a. Is an isotope of oxygen.
b. Is a paramagnetic gas.
c. Is formed by the action of ultraviolet radiation on oxygen.
d. Acts as an effective screen against ultraviolet radiations in the upper atmosphere.
e. Parts per million for parts per million is more toxic than carbon monoxide.

98　Nitrous oxide:

a. Is an endothermic compound.
b. Is a paramagnetic gas.
c. Is kinetically stable at room temperature.
d. Combines easily with water to form an acid.
e. Produces its anaesthetic effect by acting at GABA receptors.

99　The following are features associated with the behaviour of nitrous oxide:

a. Paul Bert effect.
b. Hamburger phenomenon.
c. Cushing effect.
d. Fink phenomenon.
e. Second gas effect.

100　The following gases for medical use are obtained by fractional distillation of air:

a. Oxygen.
b. Nitrogen.
c. Carbon dioxide.
d. Helium.
e. Xenon.

101　Xenon:

a. Is the only noble gas capable of acting as an anaesthetic under normobaric conditions.
b. Is present in a higher concentration in air than is argon.
c. As an anaesthetic is more potent than nitrous oxide.
d. Produces its effect by action at $GABA_A$ receptors.
e. Undergoes no known biotransformation in the body.

102   The following are higher for xenon than for nitrous oxide:

a. Molecular weight.
b. MAC.
c. Critical temperature.
d. Blood–gas partition coefficient.
e. Percentage biotransformation.

103   When compared with xenon, nitrous oxide has a:

a. Higher density.
b. Lower viscosity.
c. Higher boiling point.
d. Faster rate of anaesthetic recovery.
e. Faster rate of diffusion down the same concentration gradient.

104   Xenon:

a. Is obtained by fractional distillation of air.
b. Can be monitored by the method of infrared analysis.
c. Has a higher density than air.
d. Has a lower viscosity than oxygen.
e. Undergoes biotransformation.

105   The following activities are attributes of entonox:

a. Poynting effect.
b. Lamination.
c. Pseudo-critical temperature.
d. Fink phenomenon.
e. Paul Bert effect.

106   Helium:

a. Is obtained for medical use by fractional distillation of air.
b. Is the only gas that still remains liquid at near 0 kelvin.
c. Is found in a higher concentration in air than is argon.
d. Has a lower viscosity than nitrogen.
e. Is used as a substitute for nitrogen in breathing gas mixtures in deep sea diving primarily to minimize the effects of the 'bends' when re-surfacing.

107   Helium has a recognized role in the following:

a. Measurement of residual lung volume.
b. Working of the CO_2 laser.
c. In the management of lower airways obstruction.
d. In the functioning of the MRI scanner.
e. In the determination of the permeability of the alveolar–capillary membrane to gases.

108   Helium is the preferred substitute for nitrogen under hyperbaric conditions for the following reasons:

   a. Unlike nitrogen, helium has no detectable narcotic properties even at several atmospheres pressure.
   b. Lower solubility than nitrogen in body tissues and therefore less intensity of the 'bends' on emergence.
   c. Lesser hindrance to breathing because of its lower density compared with nitrogen.
   d. Less likely to cause hypothermia than nitrogen.
   e. Lower flammability than nitrogen and therefore reduces any fire risk.

109   The 'filling ratio' is applicable to cylinders containing the following agents:

   a. Nitrogen.
   b. Nitrous oxide.
   c. 21% O_2 in 79% helium.
   d. Air.
   e. Cyclopropane.

110   The 'filling ratio' is applicable to cylinders containing the following agents:

   a. Oxygen.
   b. Entonox.
   c. 5% CO_2 in oxygen.
   d. Helium.
   e. Carbon dioxide.

111   The following cylinders when 'full' have a gauge pressure of 137 bar:

   a. Size D oxygen cylinder.
   b. Size E nitrous oxide cylinder.
   c. Size G entonox cylinder.
   d. Size J air cylinder.
   e. Size F helium/oxygen cylinder.

112   The vapour pressure of an inhalational anaesthetic agent is dependent on:

   a. Atmospheric pressure.
   b. Ambient temperature.
   c. Boiling point of the agent.
   d. Molecular weight of the agent.
   e. Specific density of the liquid agent.

113   Parts per million for parts per million ozone is more toxic to the human body than:

   a. Carbon monoxide.
   b. Hydrogen sulphide.
   c. Hydrogen cyanide.
   d. Nitrogen dioxide.
   e. Sulphur dioxide.

114 Other things being equal, nitrous oxide will diffuse faster down a concentration gradient than:

a. Oxygen.
b. Carbon dioxide.
c. Nitric oxide.
d. Diethyl ether.
e. Xenon.

115 The following absorb infrared radiations:

a. Water vapour.
b. Oxygen.
c. Ozone.
d. Carbon dioxide.
e. CFCs (chlorofluorocarbons).

Anaesthetic machine

116 The Boyle anaesthetic machine:

a. Is named after Robert Boyle.
b. Today needs no antistatic precautions as explosive anaesthetic agents are no longer in use.
c. Delivers gases at a pressure of about 400 kPa up the flowmeter tubes.
d. Requires pressure regulators between the pipeline supply and the flowmeter unit.
e. Must necessarily have a stainless steel work top.

117 ISO specifications require that in the case of the anaesthetic machine and its accessory equipment:

a. Machine cylinder pressure gauges be inclined about 15 degrees backwards from the vertical.
b. The machine oxygen flowmeter control shall stand proud of the other flowmeter controls.
c. All controls open by being turned clockwise.
d. In the event of failure of the oxygen supply, the supply of all other gases to the flowmeter unit shall be cut off.
e. All TEC vaporizer dial faces shall be in the vertical plane.

118 The following are mandatory requirements for the modern anaesthetic machine under ISO specifications:

a. The oxygen flowmeter tube shall be at the extreme right end of the flowmeter unit.
b. The pressure gauge dials shall indicate increasing pressure in a clockwise direction.
c. The pressure gauge dial shall show the low pressure range between the 6 o'clock and 9 o'clock positions of the dial face.
d. The oxygen cut-off warning device shall have a visual alarm component.
e. All vaporizer control dials shall have their faces in the vertical plane.

119 **The oxygen cut-off warning device on the modern anaesthetic machine:**

a. Requires a supply of electricity for its proper operation.
b. Necessarily needs its own reservoir of oxygen for its correct operation.
c. When operational shall ensure that all other gases flowing up the flowmeter unit tubes are cut off at base.
d. Must when activated last for a minimum of 12 seconds in accordance with ISO specifications.
e. Must when activated produce an audible alarm of 60 decibel intensity in accordance with ISO specifications.

120 **The Bodok seal on the anaesthetic machine:**

a. Is situated 'downstream' of the pressure regulators.
b. Is usually made of neoprene.
c. Can properly be made of compressed fibre or cork.
d. Must be composed of material such that it can withstand the effects of adiabatic decompression.
e. Should not have any mineral oil in its vicinity.

121 **The flowmeter tubes in the anaesthetic machine:**

a. Work on the variable pressure differential, fixed orifice principle.
b. Are noninterchangeable in position for the different gaseous agents.
c. Are no more accurate than to within 5–6%.
d. Deliver gases along them at 400 kPa.
e. Need to be rendered antistatic even though no explosive anaesthetic agents are used today.

122 **In the modern anaesthetic machine oxygen at a pressure of 400 kPa:**

a. Flows up the flowmeter tube.
b. Energizes the oxygen cut-off warning device.
c. Provides oxygen to the 'oxygen flush'.
d. Operates the nitrous oxide cut-off valve in the event of impending failure of oxygen.
e. Is the usual 'driving gas' for the Manley MP 3 ventilator.

123 **The 'oxygen flush' on the anaesthetic machine:**

a. When activated is supplied with oxygen at a pressure of 4 bar.
b. Usually delivers oxygen at a flow rate of about 10–15 L min^{-1}.
c. Must be capable of delivering oxygen at a flow rate to match the patient's maximum breathing capacity.
d. May be allowed to be locked in the 'ON' position according to ISO specifications.
e. When operational will necessarily totally cut off oxygen flow up the oxygen flowmeter tube.

124 The following size cylinders are compatible with the modern anaesthetic machine:

a. Size C.
b. Size D.
c. Size E.
d. Size F.
e. Size G.

125 In the case of anaesthetic machine cylinders:

a. Oxygen cylinders of size F can be engaged on the pin index interface.
b. Nitrous oxide cylinders must necessarily be engaged in the vertical position.
c. Carbon dioxide cylinders can be of size E.
d. A pressure gauge on a cyclopropane cylinder gives an accurate indication of the contents of the agent.
e. All the above four types of cylinder need a pressure regulator in the gas pathway between them and the flowmeter unit.

Vaporizers

126 A 'plenum' vaporizer:

a. By definition has carrier gases passing through it at a pressure greater than atmospheric pressure.
b. Always has a temperature compensation device.
c. Has sometimes been used as a draw-over vaporizer.
d. First came into use as the 'Fluotec' vaporizer.
e. Must necessarily be heavy.

127 The following vaporizers function on the variable bypass principle:

a. Boyle bottle.
b. Desflurane vaporizer.
c. EMO vaporizer.
d. Fluotec Mark 3 vaporizer.
e. Halox vaporizer.

128 A TEC vaporizer:

a. Will deliver a higher volumes per cent of the agent at the top of Mount Everest than the dial would indicate (room temperature being the same, i.e. c. 21 °C).
b. Will deliver a higher partial pressure of the agent in a hyperbaric chamber than at standard atmospheric pressure.
c. Will deliver a higher concentration of the agent if the carrier gas is changed from N_2O/O_2 80%/20% to helium/O_2 80%/20%.
d. Will offer a lower resistance to flow in the inlet pathway under hypobaric conditions.
e. Tends to have a lower agent output at higher ambient temperatures.

129 Temperature compensation, when present with the following vaporizers, is essentially effected by provision of a 'heatsink':

a. Boyle bottle.
b. EMO vaporizer.
c. TEC Mark 3 halothane vaporizer.
d. TEC Mark 4 isoflurane vaporizer.
e. Desflurane vaporizer.

130 The isoflurane TEC Mark 4 vaporizer can correctly be called a:

a. Variable by-pass vaporizer.
b. Temperature compensated vaporizer.
c. Plenum vaporizer.
d. Concentration calibrated vaporizer.
e. High resistance vaporizer.

131 The 'pumping effect' in respect of TEC plenum anaesthetic vaporizers is more pronounced if the following are lower rather than higher:

a. Fresh gas flow rates.
b. Vaporizer dial settings.
c. Level of liquid anaesthetic in the vaporizer.
d. Ventilation rate.
e. Resistance to gas flow in gas inlet tube into vaporizing chamber.

132 The present day TEC vaporizer:

a. Is necessarily the same thing as a plenum vaporizer.
b. Has its bimetallic strip in the bypass chamber.
c. Provides its temperature compensation essentially by the provision of a large heatsink.
d. Has a long and tortuous inlet tube to the vaporizing chamber so as to minimize the 'pumping effect'.
e. Can, if required, be used effectively as a draw-over vaporizer.

133 The following statements are true with respect to anaesthetic vaporizers:

a. A variable bypass vaporizer is also a 'concentration-calibrated' vaporizer.
b. In a TEC vaporizer temperature compensation is provided primarily by the provision of a large heatsink.
c. The ISO standard for vaporizers now requires that the control dial opens counter-clockwise.
d. The ISO standard now requires that the face of the control dial shall always be in the horizontal plane.
e. A draw-over vaporizer may be usable as a plenum vaporizer, but a plenum vaporizer cannot necessarily be used as a draw-over vaporizer.

134   The Desflurane vaporizer:

a. Is rated as a 'Mark 5' vaporizer.
b. Has interlocks that prevent other vaporizers being switched on when it is in use.
c. Cannot be filled during its warm-up cycle.
d. Has a higher chamber capacity than other TEC vaporizers.
e. Its alarms and liquid crystal level indicator display are battery powered.

Ventilators

135   In the case of mechanical ventilators and their performance:

a. The Manley MP 3 will maintain a constant ventilation rate despite a change in pre-set tidal volume.
b. The Penlon 900 AV ventilator can maintain its pre-set tidal volume despite a change in the input fresh gas flow rate.
c. The Nuffield Penlon 200 ventilator can be made to deliver a tidal volume lower than the pre-set tidal volume.
d. The Pneupac ventilator can be made to deliver air alone for ventilating a patient.
e. A constant flow generator ventilator has the capacity to deliver its pre-set tidal volume irrespective of the patient's lung compliance.

136   A constant pressure generator ventilator:

a. Is necessarily a 'minute volume divider' ventilator.
b. Shows a positive accelerating exponential change with respect to the rate of gas ingress into the lungs during the inspiratory phase.
c. Can, if need be, effect full delivery of the pre-set tidal volume simply by prolonging the inspiratory time.
d. Is an appropriate ventilator for long-term IPPV of ITU patients.
e. Is exemplified by the Penlon AV 900 ventilator.

137   During IPPV using a mechanical ventilator, the peak inspiratory pressure will vary with:

a. Resistance in the ventilatory circuit.
b. Resistance of a water bath humidifier positioned in the afferent pathway of the circuit.
c. Compliance of the ventilator.
d. Patient's airway resistance.
e. Patient's static lung compliance.

138   The following are 'time-cycled flow generator' ventilators:

a. Nuffield Penlon 200 ventilator.
b. Manley MP 3 ventilator.
c. Penlon AV 600 ventilator.
d. Penlon AV 900 ventilator.
e. Ohmeda ventilator.

Equipment

139   Medical gas cylinders may properly be made of the following materials:

a. Molybdenum steel.
b. Manganese steel.
c. Carbon steel.
d. Lead.
e. Aluminium.

140   The following gas cylinders must necessarily be mounted in the vertical position for correct use:

a. Oxygen.
b. Nitrous oxide.
c. Entonox.
d. Helium/oxygen mixture.
e. 5% CO_2 in oxygen.

141   The following devices have a linear scale of graduations:

a. Anaesthetic machine oxygen flowmeter tube.
b. Wright respirometer.
c. Bourdon pressure gauge on a nitrous oxide cylinder.
d. Mercury sphygmomanometer.
e. Mercury clinical thermometer.

142   The Wright respirometer:

a. Is a variable orifice–constant pressure differential meter.
b. Is an inferential meter.
c. Can also measure flow in the reverse direction.
d. Over-reads at low tidal volumes.
e. Is available in a paediatric version.

143   The Bourdon gauge on the anaesthetic machine:

a. Is an accurate indicator of the contents of a CO_2 cylinder.
b. Has an accuracy to within 5%.
c. Shows a change in the cross-sectional configuration of its measuring tube from an ellipse to a circle with a fall in pressure inside the cylinder.
d. Must have its dial face inclined at an angle of 15 degrees to the vertical in accordance with ISO regulations.
e. Must have the low pressure graduations between the 6 o'clock and 9 o'clock positions of the dial face in accordance with ISO regulations.

144   The performance of the following devices involves gas entrainment in accordance with the Venturi effect:

a. Fixed performance oxygen mask.
b. Sanders' injector.
c. Anaesthetic machine flowmeter for the administration of air.
d. Anaesthetic machine suction apparatus operated by the piped vacuum system.
e. Suction apparatus operated by connection to an oxygen cylinder.

145   The Magill breathing attachment:

a. Is a Mapleson B attachment.
b. Is a 'semi-closed' breathing attachment.
c. When in use for spontaneous ventilation usually contains fresh gases in its 'reservoir' bag.
d. Is more efficient than the parallel Lack attachment for spontaneous ventilation.
e. Is less satisfactory for children than the co-axial Bain attachment when used in spontaneous ventilation mode.

146   When the Magill breathing attachment is used for spontaneous ventilation, a higher end-tidal CO_2 will result if:

a. If the fresh gas flow is less than the patient's alveolar ventilation.
b. If the APL valve is maintained in the 'open' position in both phases of ventilation.
c. If the length of the tubing between bag and patient is doubled with the same conventional fresh gas flow rate.
d. If a second, equal length of tubing is placed between bag and common gas outlet.
e. If the bag is detached from the bag mount.

147   The resistance to expiration during spontaneous ventilation from a Magill anaesthetic breathing attachment is greater if:

a. The fresh gas flow rate is higher.
b. The spring of the APL valve is longer.
c. The APL valve disc is broader.
d. The breathing tube is shorter.
e. If the 'reservoir bag' is removed and its attachment port is closed.

148   In the case of the co-axial Bain attachment:

a. It is a Mapleson A attachment.
b. It has an outer co-axial afferent limb.
c. It is less efficient than the Magill attachment for manual artificial ventilation ('hand bagging').
d. When used for adult spontaneous ventilation with 'standard' fresh gas flows, its breathing bag contains predominantly fresh gases.
e. Disconnection of the inner co-axial tube from the outer tube near to the patient end, during spontaneous ventilation, will lead to significant hypercapnia.

149 The Waters' to-and-fro breathing attachment:

a. Is a Mapleson E attachment.
b. When in conventional usage contains solely fresh gas in the breathing bag.
c. Can be used, suitably modified, as an anaesthetic attachment for low flow anaesthesia.
d. Suitably down-sized, can be used safely for paediatric anaesthesia in spontaneous ventilation mode.
e. Can give an FiO_2 of near 1.0 with an oxygen flow input comparable with the patient's minute volume.

150 When a patient is breathing spontaneously from the following breathing attachments with a fresh gas flow sufficient to maintain near-normocapnia, the breathing bag contains essentially fresh gases:

a. Magill attachment.
b. Bain non-co-axial attachment.
c. Bain co-axial attachment.
d. Lack attachment.
e. Parallel Lack attachment.

151 During spontaneous ventilation from the following breathing attachments there necessarily will be hypercapnia if the fresh gas flow rate is less than the patient's minute volume:

a. Magill attachment.
b. Bain co-axial attachment.
c. Parallel Lack attachment.
d. Ayre T-piece attachment with Jackson Rees modification.
e. Waters' to-and-fro breathing attachment.

152 Disconnection of the breathing bag during spontaneous ventilation from the following breathing attachments will give rise to immediate and significant hypercapnia in the patient:

a. Magill attachment.
b. Lack co-axial attachment.
c. Parallel Lack attachment.
d. Bain co-axial attachment.
e. Ayre T-piece attachment with Jackson Rees modification.

153 The reaction of soda lime with CO_2 in an anaesthetic breathing attachment:

a. Is an endothermic reaction.
b. Is normally catalyst driven.
c. Is a reversible chemical reaction.
d. Is necessarily dependent on the presence of water.
e. Leads to a net gain in water production.

154 Carbon monoxide is more likely to be produced in a low flow circle breathing attachment with soda lime if:

a. The soda lime is dry rather than moist.
b. The soda lime contains more rather than less potassium hydroxide.
c. The soda lime is hotter rather than less hot.
d. The indicator dye is clayton yellow rather than phenolphthalein.
e. Desflurane rather than isoflurane is used as the inhalational agent.

155 The following contaminants have been known to collect in a low flow circle breathing attachment with provision for CO_2 absorption during anaesthesia as a result of reaction between the inhalational anaesthetic agent and soda lime:

a. Acetone.
b. Carbon monoxide.
c. BCDFE (bromo-chloro-difluoroethylene).
d. Methane.
e. Carbonyl chloride.

156 The following are known to accumulate in a low flow breathing attachment with soda lime when sevoflurane is used as the inhalational anaesthetic agent:

a. Compound A.
b. Formic acid.
c. Methanol.
d. Formaldehyde.
e. Hexafluoropropanol.

157 The following are known to accumulate in a low flow breathing attachment with soda lime provision for CO_2 absorption when halothane is used as the inhalational anaesthetic agent:

a. Carbon monoxide.
b. Carbonyl chloride.
c. BCDFE (bromo-chloro-difluoroethylene).
d. Hexafluoropropanol.
e. Formic acid.

158 The amount of the agent contained in each of the following cylinders can be determined by application of the Universal Gas equation:

a. Oxygen cylinder.
b. Nitrous oxide cylinder.
c. Helium/oxygen 79%/21% cylinder.
d. Air cylinder.
e. Cyclopropane cylinder.

159 The following medical gas cylinders, when 'full', have a gauge pressure of about 137 bar:

a. Oxygen.
b. Entonox.
c. Air.
d. 79% helium in oxygen.
e. Carbon dioxide.

160 The following gas cylinders are available with pin index outlets:

a. Size C carbon dioxide cylinders.
b. Size D nitrous oxide cylinders.
c. Size F oxygen cylinders.
d. Size G entonox cylinders.
e. Size J oxygen cylinders.

161 The following are modifications of the Tuohy epidural needle:

a. Huber tip.
b. Murphy eye.
c. Scott hub.
d. Crawford bevel.
e. Weiss wing.

162 The following items of equipment have a 'double cuff':

a. Tourniquet used for a Bier's block.
b. Von Recklinghausen oscillotonometer used for blood pressure measurement.
c. Blood pressure cuff used with the DINAMAP.
d. Laser flex tube used for orotracheal intubation during anaesthesia for laser surgery in the throat.
e. Pallister single lumen endobronchial tube.

163 A fibre-optic light delivery system:

a. Operates on the principle of total internal reflection.
b. Needs cladding of another material with a much higher refractive index for it to be functional.
c. Must necessarily have its fibres laid coherently for its proper functioning.
d. Typically has optical fibres with a diameter of the order of 0.2 mm.
e. Can concentrate fibre light energy to the extent of it being a fire risk.

Monitoring

164   The following statements are true in respect of each of the
       following methods of gas monitoring:

   a. Mass spectrometry requires prior ionization of the sampled gases.
   b. Raman scattering is only possible if the agent for analysis
      contains at least two different elements in its molecule.
   c. In infrared gas analysis accuracy requires that water vapour be
      excluded from the sampled gases.
   d. Accurate paramagnetic analysis of oxygen requires that some
      oxides of nitrogen be absent from the sample.
   e. The Clark cell method for oxygen analysis will not be possible
      without an extraneous source of electricity.

165   The following gases can be assayed by the method of Raman
       scattering:

   a. Helium.
   b. Nitrogen.
   c. Carbon monoxide.
   d. Xenon.
   e. Oxygen.

166   The following methods of gas monitoring safely permit return of
       the sampled gases back to the patient anaesthetic breathing
       attachment:

   a. Mass spectrometry.
   b. Raman scattering.
   c. Infrared analysis.
   d. Ultraviolet analysis.
   e. Piezo-electric method

167   The presence of water vapour in the sample gas(es) will vitiate the
       accuracy of the following methods of analysis:

   a. Mass spectrometry.
   b. Paramagnetic analysis.
   c. Infrared analysis.
   d. Ultraviolet analysis.
   e. Piezo-electric crystal method.

168   Piezo-electric methods of gas analysis are applicable to
       measurement of the following:

   a. Oxygen.
   b. Halothane.
   c. Carbon dioxide.
   d. Sevoflurane.
   e. Helium.

169 **Capnography by infrared analysis:**

a. Is based on the Beer–Lambert Law.
b. Is a useful indicator of oesophageal intubation.
c. Is a reliable pointer to endobronchial intubation.
d. Can be vitiated by the presence of nitrous oxide in the gas sample.
e. Can be adversely affected by the presence of glass windows in the analyzing chamber.

170 **In gas analysis by mass spectrometry:**

a. All the commonly used anaesthetic gases can be measured by this method.
b. Gas levels are estimated in partial pressure units.
c. The analysed gas fractions can be safely returned to the patient breathing attachment.
d. The components are separated out in a trajectory that is in direct proportion to their mass:charge ratio.
e. Accurate measurement requires the mode of gas flow in the measuring chamber to be molecular rather than viscous.

171 **Infrared gas analysis:**

a. Can be used effectively for mono-atomic gases.
b. Is possible for symmetric polyatomic molecules.
c. Is an appropriate method for halogenated inhalational anaesthetic agents.
d. Should not involve return of analysed gas samples to the patient breathing circuit.
e. Provides more accurate data at higher rather than lower patient ventilation rates.

172 **The Raman scattering effect as a means of gas analysis:**

a. Is a form of 'elastic scattering'.
b. Involves a complete transfer of energy from EMRs to particles of matter.
c. Is associated with both Stokes and anti-Stokes radiations.
d. Includes Rayleigh scattering.
e. Can be applied to mono-atomic molecules.

173 **In the case of piezo-electric methods of gas analysis:**

a. They can measure oxygen.
b. They can necessarily distinguish between different halogenated inhalational anaesthetic agents.
c. They will safely allow return of monitored gas samples to patient breathing attachment.
d. Their levels of accuracy are significantly affected by the presence of water vapour in the gas sample.
e. They estimate the relevant agent by a volumes per cent method rather than a partial pressure method.

174   The following gases can be analysed by mass spectrometry:

a. Oxygen.
b. Nitrogen.
c. Helium.
d. Carbon dioxide.
e. Nitrous oxide.

175   Carbon dioxide can be assayed by the following methods of gas analysis:

a. Mass spectrometry.
b. Raman scattering.
c. Infrared gas analysis.
d. Paramagnetic analysis.
e. Piezo-electric method of gas analysis.

176   Conventional pulse oximetry:

a. Can by itself give an approximate indication of the oxygen content of blood.
b. Is a pointer, albeit indirect, to the partial pressure of oxygen in the blood.
c. Can accurately warn of one-lung ventilation.
d. Usually registers a falsely low reading in the presence of carboxyhaemoglobin.
e. Will always show a falsely low reading in the presence of methaemoglobinaemia.

177   The performance of paramagnetic oxygen analysers:

a. Is based on the presence of spin-paired electrons in the outer orbit of oxygen atoms.
b. Is affected by the presence of water vapour.
c. Is dependent on atmospheric pressure.
d. Is dependent on the production of 'magnetic wind'.
e. Is vitiated in the presence of some oxides of nitrogen.

178   The presence of the following gases in the sample mixture have been known to vitiate the accuracy of oxygen measurement by paramagnetic analysis:

a. Nitrogen.
b. Nitrous oxide.
c. Nitric oxide.
d. Nitrogen dioxide.
e. Nitrogen peroxide.

179   Nitrous oxide has been known to interfere with the following:

a. CO_2 estimation by infrared analysis.
b. Polarographic analysis of oxygen.
c. Oxygen estimation by paramagnetic analysis.
d. Measurement of halothane by ultraviolet light.
e. Isoflurane estimation by the piezo-electric method.

180 The presence of the following are known to affect the accuracy of CO_2 estimation by the method of infrared analysis:

a. Nitrous oxide.
b. Oxygen.
c. Nitrogen.
d. Glass.
e. Sapphire.

181 The presence of the following agents in the sample gas(es) is recognized as interfering with the accuracy of CO_2 estimation by infrared analysis:

a. Helium.
b. Water vapour.
c. Desflurane.
d. Cyclopropane.
e. Alcohol.

182 In the case of the Clark cell electrode method of oxygen analysis:

a. The Clark 'cell' is a voltaic cell.
b. The method measures 'volumes per cent' of oxygen.
c. A constant temperature is essential for the accuracy of the method.
d. The presence of inhalational anaesthetic agents has been known to vitiate the accuracy of the method.
e. The definitive chemical reaction is the same as in the fuel cell method of oxygen analysis.

183 The following features are common to the Clark cell and the fuel cell as methods of oxygen analysis:

a. They both have a platinum anode.
b. They both have a lead cathode.
c. Potassium is a common ion in their electrolyte solutions.
d. Need a source of electricity (a battery).
e. Common chemical reaction with oxygen.

184 The accuracy of display of an ECG signal is enhanced if the system possesses:

a. A high signal-to-noise ratio.
b. A low common mode rejection ratio.
c. A high degree of 'cross-talk'.
d. A low level of zero stability.
e. A high degree of 'polarization' at electrodes.

185 The advantages of a Ag/AgCl (silver/silver chloride) electrode include the following:

a. Less likelihood of electrolysis at electrode–skin interface.
b. Good stability.
c. Robustness.
d. Absence of photosensitivity and therefore of voltage changes.
e. Minimum noise.

186 The piezo-electric principle is an essential operative in the functioning of the following:

a. Ultrasound scanner.
b. Magnetic resonance imaging unit.
c. Invasive arterial blood pressure monitoring assembly.
d. Oxygen saturation monitor sensor diode.
e. Infrared thermometer.

Electricity and magnetism

187 A mains 'phase supply' voltage (rather than a 'line supply' voltage) in the UK:

a. Is the same as an SELV supply.
b. Has an RMS value of 240 V.
c. Is the supply more likely to be used in a radiology department than an operating theatre.
d. Cannot be used for ordinary domestic use.
e. Is the supply for operation of lifts (elevators) in a hospital.

188 The following are true with respect to electricity:

a. AC electricity is safer than DC electricity in respect of the risk of producing ventricular fibrillation.
b. The presence of a properly connected earth cable can in itself create a risk of electrocution.
c. An 'isolated' electric supply is a guarantee against electrocution.
d. Electricity is transmitted over long distances at high voltage so as to minimize energy losses during transmission.
e. A battery DC electrical source is an effective means of heating fluids.

189 High frequency alternating electric current is the basis of:

a. Transmission of mains electricity from the generating plant to electrical substations.
b. Production of the 'diathermy' current for electrosurgery.
c. Generation of ultrasound for diagnostic purposes.
d. Production of the laser beam of the CO_2 laser.
e. Heat therapy as part of physiotherapy.

190 The following necessarily need a mains (AC) supply of electricity (or an AC electricity generator), rather than a battery source, for their proper performance:

a. Penlon AV 900 ventilator.
b. Desflurane Mark 6 vaporizer.
c. Bair Hugger.
d. Fluid warmer.
e. Diathermy (electrosurgical) unit.

191 **DC rather than AC electricity is the preferred modality for operation of the following:**

a. SELV for electrical cautery (as opposed to diathermy) of skin warts.
b. Working of a defibrillator.
c. Operation of a TENS (transcutaneous electrical nerve stimulation).
d. Maintenance of magnetic field in a MRI scanner.
e. Production of continuous-wave mode during ultrasound scanning.

192 **The following need an 'external' source of electrical energy to be functional:**

a. Galvanic cell oxygen analyser.
b. Polarographic cell oxygen analyser.
c. Oxygen cut-off warning device on the anaesthetic machine.
d. Temperature determination by LCD (liquid crystal display) method.
e. Manley ventilator.

193 **The following are correct definitions of the joule:**

a. The work done when 1 coulomb of quantum of electricity is moved through a potential difference of 1 volt.
b. The energy required to make 1 ampere of current flow through a resistance of 1 ohm.
c. The energy produced when 1 watt of power is dissipated in 1 second.
d. The work done when a force of 1 newton moves an object through a distance of 1 metre.
e. The work required to move 1 cubic metre of gas against a pressure of 1 kilopascal.

194 **The duration of operational activity of each of the following is of the order of microseconds rather than milliseconds:**

a. Radiofrequency pulse during magnetic resonance imaging.
b. 'Outgoing' ultrasound pulse wave.
c. Duration of exposure during plain radiography.
d. DC shock current during manual DC cardioconversion.
e. Stimulus delivery time during use of a peripheral nerve stimulator.

195 **The voltage when the following devices are operational is in the kilovolt range:**

a. Peripheral nerve stimulator.
b. Diathermy.
c. DC defibrillator.
d. Ultrasound scanner.
e. MRI signal.

196 The mean amplitude of the following bio-electric signals is in the 1–10 mV range:

a. Electrocardiogram.
b. Electroencephalogram.
c. Electromyogram.
d. Electroretinogram.
e. Potential difference across a polarographic cell for measuring oxygen.

197 The unit of measurement of the following electrical quantities is the ohm:

a. Resistance.
b. Capacitance.
c. Inductance.
d. Impedance.
e. Reactance.

198 The predominant electrical property that determines the following activities is current:

a. Nerve stimulation by use of a peripheral nerve stimulator.
b. Cause of ventricular fibrillation in electrocution.
c. Treatment of ventricular fibrillation by manual DC cardioconversion.
d. Determination of temperature by means of a thermocouple.
e. Avoidance of thermal injury under a diathermy pad during electrosurgery.

199 Impedance in relation to electricity:

a. Is only relevant to an AC circuit.
b. Includes both *resistance* and *reactance*.
c. Has the *ohm* as its SI unit of measurement.
d. Always has a direct linear relationship with voltage.
e. Can in a circuit sometimes be equal to *resistance* alone.

200 Reactance as a form of opposition to the flow of electricity:

a. Is one type of electrical impedance.
b. Is a feature of AC circuits, only if they have a capacitor and/or inductor in them.
c. Is measured in ohms.
d. Always increases with increasing frequency of the AC current.
e. Is denoted by the symbol Z.

201 Reactance as a form of opposition to the flow of electric current is possible in the following:

a. A DC circuit with only a resistor.
b. A DC circuit with a resistor and a capacitor.
c. A DC circuit with a resistor and an inductor.
d. An AC circuit with a resistor, capacitor and an inductor.
e. An AC circuit with a capacitor and an inductor.

202   The following are associated with the phenomenon of magnetism:

a. Boyle temperature.
b. Transition temperature.
c. Curie temperature.
d. Neel temperature.
e. Critical temperature.

203   Paramagnetism:

a. Is stronger than diamagnetism.
b. Is a property present only in elements possessing unpaired electrons.
c. Is demonstrated by materials having negative (magnetic) susceptibility.
d. Is associated with the presence of magnetic domains.
e. Is exhibited by nitric oxide.

204   In the case of diamagnetism:

a. It is a property present in all substances.
b. It is unaffected by temperature.
c. It possesses a relative permeability of slightly more than one.
d. It is associated with the property of coercivity.
e. Its magnetization susceptibility is negative.

205   Ferromagnetism:

a. Is temperature dependent.
b. Is associated with the presence of magnetic 'domains' in its materials.
c. Is susceptible to 'saturation'.
d. Possesses the attribute of remanence.
e. Is prone to hysteresis.

206   The 'diathermy plate' can correctly be called the following:

a. Dispersive electrode plate.
b. Earthing plate.
c. Grounding plate.
d. Indifferent electrode plate.
e. Return electrode plate.

207   The use of a 'REM' (return electrode monitoring) diathermy plate:

a. Is only possible with an 'isolated' diathermy (electrosurgical) unit.
b. Will help reduce the likelihood of thermal injury of the skin under the plate.
c. Is necessary if the cutting mode of diathermy is being used.
d. Is unnecessary if bipolar diathermy is being used.
e. Is necessary if the diathermy switch is hand-operated rather than foot-operated.

208 The following phenomena are related to the activity of diathermy (electrosurgery):

a. Crest factor.
b. Duty cycle.
c. Cavitation.
d. Channelling.
e. Free induction decay.

209 'Resonant frequency' is a relevant phenomenon in relation to the working of the following devices:

a. Fluid coupled transducer in invasive arterial blood pressure monitoring.
b. Production of laser light beam in the CO_2 laser.
c. Use of the MRI scanner in imaging.
d. Production of an ultrasound wave by the piezo-electric crystal of an ultrasound unit.
e. Activity of the phosphor in the element of a fluorescent strip light.

210 The following can be made to perform their function without a supply of electrical energy:

a. The Manley ventilator.
b. The Nuffield Penlon 200 ventilator.
c. A liquid crystal thermometer.
d. An infrared thermometer.
e. A suction apparatus attached to an anaesthetic machine.

211 The following phenomena are essential prerequisites for the proper functioning of a DC defibrillator:

a. Rectification.
b. Inductance.
c. Remanence
d. Capacitance.
e. Population inversion.

212 High electrical impedance (resistance) is a necessary requirement for the following:

a. Antistatic theatre footwear.
b. Antistatic theatre flooring.
c. Mains protective earth cabling.
d. ECG skin electrodes.
e. Electrodes for use of PNS (peripheral nerve stimulator).

213 The following statements are true:

a. Class I electrical equipment possesses a protective earth cable.
b. Class II electrical equipment has no symbol.
c. Class III electrical equipment is low-voltage equipment.
d. Type CF electrical equipment has a higher maximum permitted leakage current under single fault conditions than do BF equipment.
e. Use of 'isolated' electrical equipment eliminates the likelihood of electrocution.

214   The following types of electrical equipment have no designated definitive symbol of recognition in accordance with IEC (International Electrotechnical Commision) regulations:

a. Class I.
b. Class II.
c. Class III.
d. 'Anaesthetic proof' equipment.
e. Diathermy equipment that is 'isolated' at high frequency.

215   The following statements are true:

a. Class I equipment is 'doubly insulated'.
b. Class II equipment does not have a protective earth cable.
c. APG equipment is designed to provide protection against the most flammable mixture of ether and air.
d. SELV equipment may be energized by a battery DC supply.
e. 'Defibrillation proof' equipment is so labelled because it will not induce VF in patients during their use.

216   A capacitor is now a recognized component in the workings of the following items of equipment:

a. A diathermy (electrosurgical) unit.
b. A DC defibrillator.
c. A fluid coupled invasive arterial blood pressure monitoring transducer.
d. A CO_2 laser.
e. Ultrasound scanner.

217   The following are necessary components of a mains powered DC defibrillator:

a. Oscillator.
b. Rectifier.
c. Transformer.
d. Inductor.
e. Capacitor.

218   In the following phenomena the pertinent subatomic particle is the electron:

a. Flow of an electric current in a circuit.
b. Production of an ECG wave display in a cathode ray tube.
c. Production of the signal in nuclear magnetic resonance imaging.
d. Production of an X-ray image.
e. Production of a beam of laser light.

219   The following are related to magnetic resonance imaging:

a. Fink phenomenon.
b. Cannizzaro reaction.
c. Larmor frequency.
d. Peltier effect.
e. Raman scattering.

220   Hydrogen is the most commonly imaged element in magnetic resonance imaging because:

    a. It is the most abundant element in the human body.
    b. It is the lightest element.
    c. It has no isotopes.
    d. It is capable of forming hydrogen bonds.
    e. It gives the strongest MRI signal.

221   The piezo-electric effect is a phenomenon associated with:

    a. Invasive arterial blood pressure monitoring.
    b. Nuclear magnetic resonance imaging.
    c. Ultrasound diagnostic investigation.
    d. Fibre-optic transmission.
    e. Transmission of laser light energy.

222   Uses of the cathode ray oscilloscope include the following:

    a. Display of waveforms.
    b. Measurement of AC electricity voltage.
    c. Measurement of DC electricity voltage.
    d. Measurement of EMR frequencies.
    e. Measurement of small time intervals.

223   The following relate electrical activity with its heating effect:

    a. Joule effect.
    b. Thomson effect.
    c. Joule–Kelvin effect.
    d. Seebeck effect.
    e. Peltier effect.

Miscellaneous

224   The atomic number of an element:

    a. Is unique for each element.
    b. Is a dimensionless entity.
    c. Indicates the element's numbered position in the periodic table.
    d. Is equal to the number of electrons in a neutral atom.
    e. Is indicative of the isotope status of the element in question.

225   The atomic mass number:

    a. Is a dimensionless entity.
    b. May also be referred to as the element's nucleon number.
    c. Is equal to the number of electrons in a neutral atom.
    d. By convention is denoted by the symbol Z.
    e. Is the same for different isotopes of the same element.

226 In respect of bonds and secondary forces between atoms and molecules:

a. All molecules possess London forces.
b. Hydrogen bonding is present only in and between molecules containing O–H bonds.
c. Dipole–dipole forces are stronger than hydrogen bonds.
d. The presence of van der Waals forces is an essential requirement for an 'ideal gas' to conform to the gas laws.
e. The strongest bonds are ionic bonds.

227 van der Waals forces:

a. Are permanent dipole–dipole attractions.
b. Are strong forces.
c. Are present in all substances.
d. Are necessary forces for converting gases into liquids by condensation.
e. Are more likely in branched-chain compounds than in straight-chain compounds.

228 London forces are:

a. Present in all molecules.
b. Permanent dipole forces.
c. Stronger than hydrogen bonds.
d. The weakest of all van der Waals forces.
e. Stronger in larger molecule substances than smaller molecule substances.

229 Hydrogen bonding:

a. Can only form between identical molecules.
b. Is only possible between hydrogen and oxygen.
c. Accounts for the lower density of ice compared with that of water.
d. Accounts for the higher boiling point of water compared with those of other common liquids.
e. Plays a role in body temperature regulation by evaporation.

230 Hydrogen bonds:

a. Are weak dipole–dipole attractions.
b. Are stronger than London forces.
c. Occur between the bases of DNA chains.
d. Are responsible for the secondary structure of proteins.
e. Account for the high dielectric constant of water.

231 Hydrogen bonds:

a. Help determine the globular shape of proteins.
b. Provide stability to the DNA double helix.
c. Are responsible for the abnormally low vapour pressure of water.
d. Help bond 2,3-DPG (di-phosphoglycerate) to reduced haemoglobin.
e. Account for the bacterial disinfectant properties of alcohols.

232 Covalent bonds:

    a. Are the strongest of chemical bonds and molecular interactions.
    b. Involve electron transfer between donor and recipient atoms.
    c. May impart polarity to a molecule.
    d. Are the common bonds for the alkylating effect of drugs.
    e. Play a role in faithful replication of DNA.

233 The following occur by covalent bonding:

    a. Inactivation of cyclo-oxygenase by aspirin.
    b. Neutralization of heparin by protamine.
    c. Oxygenation of haemoglobin by combination with its ferrous iron moiety.
    d. Chemical reaction involved in immunogenic halothane hepatitis arising from fluoroacetylated byproducts of halothane.
    e. Binding of edrophonium to acetylcholinesterase.

234 The following statements are true:

    a. An 'ideal' gas has no van der Waals forces acting on its molecules.
    b. An 'ideal' fluid is one that behaves in accordance with the Hagen–Poiseuille equation.
    c. An 'ideal' solution conforms to Raoult's Law.
    d. A 'Newtonian' fluid has a viscosity that changes with its applied shear rate.
    e. A 'non-Newtonian' fluid has a shear rate that is independent of its velocity of flow.

235 The following are correct descriptions of 'transition temperature':

    a. The temperature at which one crystalline form of a substance changes to another form.
    b. The temperature at which a gas most closely approximates to an ideal gas.
    c. The temperature at which an electrical conductor acquires superconducting properties.
    d. The temperature at which a cell membrane changes from 'gel' form to 'sol' form or vice versa.
    e. The temperature at which a metal loses its ferromagnetic quality and becomes merely paramagnetic.

236 The following are instances of 'transition temperature':

    a. Boyle temperature.
    b. Curie temperature.
    c. Neel temperature.
    d. Colour temperature.
    e. Critical temperature.

237 The following are colligative properties:

    a. Osmolarity.
    b. Specific density.
    c. Cryoscopic constant.
    d. Vapour pressure.
    e. Thermal conductivity.

238 **The following refer to the same thing:**

a. Boyle's Law and Mariotte's Law.
b. Ionic bond and electrovalent bond.
c. Dielectric constant and relative permittivity.
d. Illuminance and intensity of illumination.
e. *Cis–trans* isomerism and dynamic isomerism.

239 **The following refer to the same thing:**

a. Poynting effect and overpressure effect.
b. Bernoulli phenomenon and Venturi effect.
c. Fink phenomenon and diffusion hypoxia.
d. Earth-free electrical circuit and floating electrical circuit.
e. Joule–Kelvin principle and Joule–Thomson effect.

240 **Isomers necessarily have:**

a. An identical elemental composition.
b. The same chemical formula.
c. The same molecular weight.
d. The same structural configuration.
e. The same atomic connectivity.

241 **The following refer to the same thing:**

a. *Structural* isomerism and *constitutional* isomerism.
b. D-, L-isomers and *d*-, *l*-isomers.
c. R-, S-configuration and the Cahn–Ingold–Prelog system.
d. *Configuration* and *conformation*.
e. Conformers and rotamers.

242 **The following statements are true:**

a. A *racemic* mixture is optically active.
b. *Cis–trans* isomerism is only possible in compounds possessing a carbon–carbon double bond (C=C).
c. Enantiomers differ from one another only in respect of chirality.
d. R-configuration agents are necessarily dextro-rotatory.
e. Diastereomers are stereo-isomers which are not mirror images of one another.

243 **The following are chiral properties:**

a. Direction of rotation of plane polarized light.
b. Degree (magnitude) of rotation of polarized light.
c. Solubility in an achiral solvent.
d. Specific density.
e. Melting point.

244   *Cis–trans* isomerism:

a. Is also known as geometric isomerism.
b. Is a feature of enantiomers.
c. Necessarily requires a carbon–carbon double bond (C=C) in the isomers concerned.
d. Necessarily implies *configuration* differences between the isomers.
e. Is a feature associated with the activity of thiopentone sodium.

245   Diastereomers may differ from one another with respect to the following properties:

a. Direction of rotation of polarized light.
b. Solubility in an achiral solvent.
c. Specific density.
d. Boiling point.
e. Melting point.

246   The enantiomers of an enantiomeric pair differ in respect of the following properties:

a. Boiling point.
b. Solubility.
c. Molecular weight.
d. Direction of rotation of plane-polarized light.
e. Degree of rotation of plane-polarized light.

247   A racemic mixture:

a. Consists of two structural isomers.
b. Must necessarily consist of chiral agents.
c. Is simply a mixture of an R- and an S-isomer.
d. Can be a mixture of two stereo-isomers.
e. Possesses optical activity.

248   The following statements are true:

a. Keto-enol tautomerism is a form of stereo-isomerism.
b. *Cis–trans* isomerism is the same as dynamic isomerism.
c. Stereo-isomers possess the same atomic connectivity but different configurational forms.
d. Enantiomers differ from one another only in respect of chirality.
e. Enflurane and isoflurane are stereo-isomers of each other.

249   The following statements are true:

a. A stereo-isomer is necessarily an *enantiomer*.
b. *Cis–trans* isomerism is necessarily a form of stereo-isomerism.
c. A (R) configuration compound is necessarily dextro-rotatory.
d. Isomers necessarily have the same atomic mass number.
e. Diastereomers necessarily differ in respect of all physical properties.

250   The following are only possible in the case of stereo-isomers:

a. *Cis–trans* isomerism.
b. Lactam–lactim isomerism.
c. Rotamerism.
d. Constitutional isomerism.
e. Configurational isomerism.

251   The fatty acids that form part of the structure of cell membranes:

a. Are all unsaturated fatty acids.
b. Usually possess an even number of carbon atoms.
c. Most commonly contain a number of carbon atoms in their teens (13 to 19).
d. Are usually *cis* in form.
e. Are almost invariably unbranched.

252   The following are the opposites or the reciprocals of each other:

a. Resistance (to fluid flow in a conduit) and compliance.
b. Resistance (to the flow of electricity in a circuit) and conductance.
c. Joule–Thomson effect and Joule–Kelvin effect.
d. Joule effect and Peltier effect.
e. Haldane effect and Bohr effect.

253   The following refer to the same thing:

a. Keto-enol tautomerism and geometric isomerism.
b. Ohm and siemens.
c. Dalton and atomic mass unit.
d. Absolute temperature scale and thermodynamic temperature scale.
e. Quetelet index and body mass index.

254   The following refer to the same thing:

a. Stress-relaxation and latch phenomenon.
b. Amphiphilicity and amphipathicity.
c. Amphotericity and amphibolicity.
d. Luminance and illuminance.
e. R-, S-isomerism and *d*-, *l*-isomerism.

255   The osmolarity of a solution is related to the following:

a. Number of solute particles per unit volume of solvent.
b. Mass of each particle of solute.
c. Number of charges per unit particle of solute.
d. Degree of dissociation of the solute.
e. Valency of each solute particle.

256 The following statements are true:

a. The SI unit of *energy* is the same as that for *heat*.
b. The units of *pressure* are the same as those of *stress*.
c. In relation to the lung, the units of *compliance* are the same as those of *conductance*.
d. The units for *illuminance* are the same as those for *luminance*.
e. *Dynamic viscosity* has the same units as *kinematic viscosity*.

257 The following are 'greenhouse gases':

a. Carbon dioxide.
b. Water.
c. Nitrogen.
d. Nitrous oxide.
e. Halothane.

258 The following statements are true:

a. The pressure inside a full oxygen cylinder is approximately 137 bar, no matter the size of the cylinder.
b. Entonox cylinders are available with pin-index heads, no matter the cylinder size.
c. The temperature inside the vaporizing chamber of a TEC vaporizer remains constant, no matter how long the vaporizer has been in use.
d. The boiling point of a liquid remains the same, no matter the ambient pressure.
e. The degree of in vivo dissociation of a polar drug remains approximately the same, no matter the plasma pH.

259 'Conductive' gel is used in the following situations to minimize electrical impedance:

a. Attachment of electrodes for electrocardiography.
b. On defibrillator pads for cardioconversion.
c. On a diathermy pad forming part of the return electrode plate.
d. On an ultrasound probe prior to ultrasound scanning.
e. Nerve stimulator electrodes when used for testing for return of neuromuscular transmission.

260 The following statements are true:

a. The higher the frequency of an alternating current, the less the opposition to its passage through an inductor.
b. The higher the frequency of an ultrasound wave, the easier its propagation through its medium of transmission.
c. The higher the frequency of electromagnetic radiations, the lower their mutagenicity.
d. The higher the resonant frequency of a fluid-coupled transducer, the lower the damping coefficient of the system.
e. The higher the frequency of a diathermy (electrosurgical unit) current, the lower the risk of thermal injury.

261 The following are graded according to FCG (French catheter gauge):

a. Nasopharyngeal airways.
b. Robertshaw double lumen tubes.
c. Epidural catheters.
d. Tracheostomy tubes.
e. Whitecare spinal needles.

262 The following are graded according to FCG (French catheter gauge):

a. Magill orotracheal tubes.
b. Mallinckrodt 'laser-flex' tubes.
c. Carlen double lumen tubes.
d. Macintosh laryngoscope blades.
e. Brain laryngeal mask airways.

263 The following are graded according to SWG (steel wire gauge):

a. Nasopharyngeal airways.
b. Hypodermic needles.
c. Intravenous cannulae.
d. Quadruple lumen central venous catheters.
e. Tuohy epidural needles.

264 The following devices incorporate a 'Murphy eye':

a. Orotracheal tubes.
b. Nasopharyngeal airways.
c. Urinary catheters.
d. Tuohy epidural needles.
e. Intravenous cannulae.

265 The following statements are true:

a. An *adiabatic* change will render Boyle's Law invalid.
b. An *isothermal* change is a necessary pre-requisite for Charles' Law to be true.
c. An *exponential* change is a valid manifestation in relation to Gay-Lussac's Law.
d. An *iso-piestic* change is an essential requirement in the behaviour of a fluid coupled transducer during invasive arterial blood pressure monitoring.
e. An *iso-volumic* change occurs during the early phase of ventricular diastole.

266 A decrease in potential energy results:

a. When a gas is compressed.
b. When a spring unwinds.
c. When the fluid flow rate in a conduit increases.
d. When an object falls from a height.
e. When a gas undergoes adiabatic decompression.

267 The figure of 'one million' (10^6) indicates:

a. The number of dynes per square centimetre pressure units roughly equal to 1 atmosphere pressure.
b. The approximate number of pascals in a bar.
c. Number of angstroms per millimetre length.
d. Number of millilitres in 1 cubic metre.
e. Frequency of the 'interrogation current' of an REM (return electrode monitoring) diathermy plate.

268 The figure of 'one hundred thousand' (10^5) indicates:

a. Number of pascals in 1 standard atmosphere pressure.
b. Number of centilitres in a cubic metre.
c. Number of dynes equal to a newton.
d. Number of dynes per square centimetre equivalent to 1 kilopascal.
e. Number of angstrom in a picometre.

269 The figure of 'one thousand' (10^3) indicates:

a. Number of centimetres water pressure equivalent to 1 atmosphere pressure.
b. Number of gauss per tesla.
c. Number of millimoles of sodium bicarbonate in a litre of 8.4% $NaHCO_3$ solution.
d. Number of torr in 1 bar.
e. Number of litres in a cubic metre.

270 The figure of 'one hundred' (10^2) indicates:

a. Number of kilopascals in 1 bar.
b. Number of rads in 1 gray.
c. Number of rems in 1 sievert.
d. Number of angstroms per nanometre.
e. Number of centimetres water pressure equivalent to 1 kilopascal.

271 The figure of 'ten' (10) indicates:

a. Number of poise (non-SI unit of dynamic viscosity) equivalent to 1 pascal second (SI unit of dynamic viscosity).
b. Number of metres water pressure equal to a pressure of 1 atmosphere.
c. Number of centimetres water pressure equal to 1 millimetre mercury pressure.
d. Number of picometres equal to 1 angstrom.
e. Number of milligrams of solute in 1 millilitre of a 1% solution.

272 The following are in the 'kilo' range rather than in the 'mega' range or higher:

a. Impedance of dry skin in ohms.
b. Voltage of transmission of AC electricity over long distances.
c. EMR frequency of a microwave oven.
d. AC frequency of the 'interrogation current' passing through an REM plate in a diathermy (electrosurgical) circuit.
e. Impedance of antistatic footwear and theatre flooring.

273 The following measuring devices indicate gauge pressure and not absolute pressure:

a. Mercury sphygmomanometer.
b. Bourdon gauge on an anaesthetic machine.
c. Mercury manometer with a Torricellian vacuum.
d. Anaeroid sphygmomanometer.
e. 'Open' CVP manometer.

274 'Resonant frequency' is a pertinent phenomenon in the performance of the following devices:

a. Fluid coupled transducer for invasive arterial blood pressure monitoring.
b. AC electrical circuit containing a capacitor and an inductor.
c. Magnetic resonance imaging.
d. Piezo-electric crystal of an ultrasound scanner.
e. Use of diathermy (electrosurgery) in the 'cutting' mode.

275 A relative humidity of 40–60% of the theatre environment is advisable:

a. For the physical comfort of theatre staff.
b. If explosive anaesthetic agents are being used.
c. To prevent build up of static electricity.
d. To effectively minimize body heat loss from patient.
e. To render safe the use of diathermy (electrosurgery).

276 The following statements are true:

a. The relationship between current and resistance in an ohmic circuit when graphically represented is in the form of a rectangular hyperbola.
b. The relationship between specific gravity (specific density) of urine and its osmolarity is always linear.
c. The viscosity of blood in vivo shows no change in the different parts of the circulation.
d. Light in its propagation always obeys the inverse square law.
e. Ice owes its lower specific density, compared with water, to the presence of hydrogen bonds.

277 The following can be properly operational without the need for a mains AC electricity supply or an AC supply such as that provided by a generator:

a. Desflurane vaporizer: maintenance of the correct pre-set anaesthetic agent concentration.
b. Penlon 600 ventilator: delivery of anaesthetic gases into patient.
c. Nuffield Penlon 200 ventilator: pre-setting of tidal volume and ventilation rate.
d. Suction apparatus on an anaesthetic machine.
e. Electrocautery for cauterization of skin warts.

278 **The following statements are true:**

a. A plenum vaporizer is necessarily a TEC vaporizer.
b. A platinum resistance thermometer necessarily involves the Wheatstone bridge principle.
c. A pressure generator ventilator is necessarily a 'minute volume divider'.
d. A DC defibrillator assembly must necessarily have a diode (rectifier) incorporated into its circuitry.
e. A Waters to-and-fro breathing attachment must necessarily be a non-return (fresh gas) flow attachment.

279 **The following statements are true:**

a. A battery operated defibrillator assembly must necessarily have an oscillator in its circuit.
b. A pipe line oxygen supply to an anaesthetic machine must necessarily have a pressure regulator between it and the flowmeter unit.
c. An intravenous fluid warmer device must necessarily incorporate a stepdown transformer in its electrical pathway.
d. A TEC Mark 4 anaesthetic vaporizer must necessarily be provided with a large heatsink.
e. Electrical cautery of tissues, as opposed to diathermy, necessarily needs a SELV electricity supply.

280 **In the following instances there is a conversion of potential energy into kinetic energy:**

a. Filling of a helium cylinder at the industrial plant.
b. Inflation of a bicycle tyre tube.
c. Unwinding of the coiled spring of a watch.
d. Performance of a 'fixed performance' oxygen mask.
e. Fluid coupled invasive arterial blood pressure measuring transducer.

281 **'Channelling' is a phenomenon associated with the following:**

a. Use of monopolar diathermy during an orchidopexy.
b. Ultrasound imaging of solid tissue.
c. Use of soda lime in a low flow anaesthetic breathing attachment for CO_2 absorption.
d. Behaviour of monopolar diathermy in a patient with a cardiac pacemaker in situ.
e. Activity of hydrogen protons when subject to a magnetic field.

282 **Coherence in relation to wave transmission is a necessary feature for the correct performance of the following:**

a. Laser light.
b. Diathermy (electrosurgery).
c. MRI.
d. Fibre-optic transmission of an image.
e. Activity of the piezo-electric crystal of an ultrasound scanner.

283 The following systems or devices normally utilize a gas pressure of 4 bar for their performance:

   a. Sanders injector used for lung ventilation during rigid bronchoscopy.
   b. Operation of nitrous oxide cut-off valve in the event of oxygen failure on the anaesthetic machine.
   c. Operation of a suction apparatus by means of a cylinder supply of oxygen.
   d. Inflation of a patient tourniquet using a pipeline supply of air.
   e. Operation of 'machine pressure relief valve' on the back bar of an anaesthetic machine.

284 The following forms of magnetism are unaffected by temperature:

   a. Paramagnetism.
   b. Diamagnetism.
   c. Ferromagnetism.
   d. Ferrimagnetism.
   e. Antiferromagnetism.

285 The following are reciprocals of one another:

   a. Frequency and wavelength in respect of EMRs.
   b. Resistance and compliance in relation to gas movement in the respiratory system.
   c. Resistance and conductance in relation to flow of electricity in a circuit.
   d. Dielectric constant and relative permittivity.
   e. Permeability and coercivity in relation to magnetism.

286 Gamma rays:

   a. Are positively charged entities.
   b. Are more energetic than X-rays.
   c. Travel at the speed of light.
   d. Have a strong ability to produce fluorescence.
   e. Obey the inverse square law in respect of intensity and distance of propagation.

287 An incorrectly higher than normal reading has been recognized as a possibility in the following situations:

   a. A haemoglobin SpO_2 saturation value during pulse oximetry in the presence of carbon monoxide.
   b. An end-tidal CO_2 reading on infrared analysis in the presence of nitrous oxide.
   c. A volumes per cent reading for an anaesthetic gas in the presence of a 'rogue' gas during gas analysis by mass spectrometry.
   d. Cardiac muscle depolarization voltage on ECG in the presence of high impedance at skin-electrode interface.
   e. A value for oxygen percentage on paramagnetic analysis in the presence of nitric oxide.

288 At very low temperatures (such as 4 kelvin):

a. Liquid helium has no viscosity.
b. Mercury loses all its electrical resistance.
c. Oxygen becomes magnetic.
d. A gas (if still in the gaseous phase) has near-zero internal energy.
e. The electron band energy structure of a semiconductor is similar to that of an insulator.

289 In a vacuum:

a. Transmission of heat energy is not possible.
b. Light waves have the highest speed of propagation.
c. Sound waves cannot be transmitted.
d. Magnetism cannot exert its effect.
e. Capacitor plates have the lowest dielectric constant.

290 The following have an inverse relationship:

a. Wavelength of peak emission of EMRs from a black body radiator and their temperature.
b. Frequency of AC electricity and reactance of a capacitor in the circuit.
c. Frequency of EMRs and their energy levels.
d. Frequency of sound waves and their degree of penetration.
e. Wavelength of ultrasound and their degree of resolution.

291 The following have a direct relationship:

a. Angular frequency of precessing protons and the static magnetic field they are subjected to during MRI.
b. Michaelis constant (K_m) of an enzyme and enzyme's affinity for its substrate.
c. Frequency of AC electricity and reactance of an inductor in the circuit.
d. Density and viscosity of a liquid.
e. Blood–gas partition coefficient of an inhalational anaesthetic agent and speed of anaesthetic induction with that agent.

292 The following show a 'square wave' pattern on graphical display:

a. PNS (peripheral nerve stimulator) on TOF (Train-of-Four) stimulation.
b. Diathermy (electrosurgical) current in cutting mode.
c. Energy discharge from a DC defibrillator during manual DC cardioconversion.
d. Waveform of ultrasound beam during a scan.
e. RF (radiofrequency) signal during magnetic resonance imaging.

293 The following show a 'square wave' pattern on graphical display:

a. Coagulation current of a diathermy (electrosurgical) unit.
b. Implanted cardiac pacemaker stimulation current.
c. Current stimulus of a TENS (transcutaneous electrical stimulation) machine.
d. Light wave of a CO_2 laser.
e. Electrical stimulus during ECT shock.

294 **The following statements are true:**

a. Temperature is the only base quantity (in the SI units system) that is not 'extensive'.
b. Radiation is the only heat transfer process that can occur in a vacuum.
c. Helium is the only gas that is still capable of existing in liquid form at near 0 kelvin.
d. Oxygen is the only paramagnetic gas that is met with in significant concentrations in clinical practice.
e. Halothane is the only halogenated inhalation anaesthetic agent that can be measured by ultraviolet analysis.

295 **The following statements are true:**

a. An *ionic* drug is charged or uncharged, depending on its environmental pH.
b. A *nonpolar* substance is incapable of assuming a charge, no matter its environmental pH.
c. A *polar* compound is permanently charged, whatever its environmental pH.
d. A *covalent* bond always possesses absolute electro-equivalence.
e. *Van der Waals forces* are strong dipole–dipole attractions.

296 **The following are correct descriptions of Curie temperature:**

a. Temperature above which a piezo-electric transducer loses its piezo-electric property.
b. Temperature below which a metal becomes electrically superconductive.
c. Temperature at which a non-ideal gas most closely approximates to an ideal gas.
d. Temperature above which a ferromagnetic material loses its ferromagnetic property.
e. Temperature above which a gas cannot be liquefied by pressure alone.

297 **A gas flow restrictor is regarded as a necessary device between:**

a. Anaesthetic machine pressure regulator ('Adams valve') and flowmeter unit.
b. Anaesthetic machine pipe line oxygen supply and flowmeter unit.
c. Ventilator driving gas (oxygen) supply and Penlon AV 900 ventilator bellows.
d. Anaesthetic machine back bar and common gas outlet.
e. Common gas outlet of anaesthetic machine and Manley MP 3 ventilator.

298 **Larmor frequency:**

a. Is an operating factor in magnetic resonance imaging.
b. Relates to precessing electrons.
c. Is in the radiofrequency range.
d. Depends only on the size of the applied magnetic field.
e. Is a factor in determining the gyro-magnetic ratio.

299 The following gauges are scaled in an anticlockwise direction:

a. Bourdon gauge of an oxygen cylinder.
b. Concentration dial of a sevoflurane vaporizer.
c. Bourdon gauge for gas pressure in the circle anaesthetic breathing circuit.
d. 'Negative pressure' gauge on a vacuum suction pipeline.
e. End-inspiratory pressure gauge of the Manley MP 3 ventilator.

300 The following are phenomena associated with the behaviour of laser light:

a. Cavitation.
b. Channelling.
c. Collimation.
d. Population inversion.
e. Precession.

301 The following relate to the activity of ultrasound imaging:

a. Acoustic impedance.
b. Superconductivity.
c. Coherence.
d. Graded index transmission.
e. Gyromagnetic ratio.

302 Ultrasound:

a. Is a form of electromagnetic radiations.
b. Shows better resolution the higher its frequency.
c. Has greater penetrative powers at longer wavelengths.
d. Has an energy level linearly proportional to the amplitude of its waves.
e. Can cause heating of tissues.

303 The following are phenomena associated with ultrasound imaging:

a. Thermal jostling.
b. Acoustic mismatch.
c. Coercivity.
d. Intensity reflection coefficient.
e. Spin–spin interaction.

304 The following relate to fibre-optic light transmission:

a. Step index transmission.
b. Coherence.
c. Remanence.
d. Spin-lattice relaxation.
e. Collimation.

1   Answers

a. False – about 1960.

b. False – it has a nongravitational basis. This was one reason for the SI units to move away from one based on a gravitational system.

c. True.

d. False – it is based on the MKSA system (metre – kilogram – second – ampere), but it does incorporate the cgs system.

e. False – the angstrom is 10^{-10} m and is equal to 0.1 nm. The SI convention is that fractions and multiples of all units shall be expressed by means of exponents of multiples of 3 and –3.

2   Answers

a. False – there are seven base quantities.

b. False – temperature is the odd one out; it is not an *extensive* quantity. An extensive property is one whose magnitude depends on the amount of the substance present in a given thermodynamic state. A more meaningful explanation is as follows: if two masses, say 3 kg and 5 kg, are put together their combined mass will be 8 kg, i.e. the sum of the individual masses. The same applies to all the other base quantities except temperature. In the case of temperature, if two fluids at respectively 20 °C and 30 °C are mixed together their 'combined' temperature will *not* be 50 °C, the sum of their individual temperatures, but an intermediate value. Therefore temperature is not an extensive quantity.

c. False – the metre is now (since 1983) defined with reference to the speed of light in a vacuum, which is 299,792,458 m s^{-1}. Therefore the metre is that distance travelled by light in a vacuum in 1/299 792 458th of a second.

d. False – it is *intensity of illumination. Luminance* (and *illuminance*) are different from intensity of illumination. *Luminance* is a measure of the luminous intensity of a surface in a given direction per unit of projected area. It refers to the effectiveness of a given light on the eye, regardless of its origin, and is a physical measure of brightness. Its unit is candela per square metre (cd m^{-2}). *Illuminance* is a measure of the quantity of light striking a surface such as a desk top or a surgical operation site. It is expressed in lumens per square metre (lm m^{-2}) or lux (lx) where 1 lx is 1 lm m^{-2}. Therefore, luminance = illuminance $\times$ reflectance, where reflectance is the amount of light emanating from a surface as a proportion of light incident on it

e. False – defined by reference to carbon-12.

3   Answers

a. False – all names of units, including those named after persons, when written in full shall commence with a lower case letter, e.g. 'pascal' not 'Pascal'.

b. True – when abbreviated, an eponymous unit shall be represented by an upper case letter, e.g. 'N' for newton, the unit of force; 'Hz' for hertz, the unit of frequency.

c. True – e.g. '100 kilograms' shall be indicated as '100 kg'.

d. False – no punctuation marks shall be used.

e. False – the abbreviation is 'm'. 'M' is the abbreviation for 'mega' as in megahertz: 'MHz'.

4   Answers

a. **False** – the correct abbreviation is 'dB'. The (upper case) B denotes 'bel', the unit of sound intensity, named after Alexander Graham Bell (1847–1922) inventor of the telephone. The more common unit is the decibel which is equal to one-tenth of a bel. 'Db' is the symbol for dubnium, one of the radioactive transactinide elements, i.e. elements with an atomic number greater than 103.

b. **False** – kilopascals is denoted as 'kPa'.

c. **False** – the correct unit is 10^3 millilitres or 10^{-3} cubic metres. The litre is a unit that is so commonly used that it has been 'adopted' as an unofficial SI unit. It was originally defined as the volume of 1 kg of pure water at 4 °C and 1 standard atmosphere pressure, which is equivalent to 1.000028 cubic decimetres.

d. **False** – the correct notation is '273 kelvin'. As the kelvin scale is an absolute scale, there are no 'degrees' in it.

e. **False** – G stands for giga; Gy is the symbol for absorbed dose of radiation.

5   Answers

a. **False** – the abbreviation is Ci; Cu stands for copper.

b. **False** – the abbreviation is Bq; B is the abbreviation for 'bel', the unit of sound intensity; see **4a**.

c. **True** – note: Z is also the symbol for electrical impedance.

d. **False** – the symbol is Z (see **5c**); R is the symbol for electrical resistance.

e. **False** – it is Sv. The abbreviation S is for siemens, the SI unit of electrical conductance.

6   Answers

a. **False** – the correct notation is 25 Hz.

b. **False** – it should be written as 10^3 m or 1 km.

c. **False** – 10^3 ml (millilitres) or 10^{-3} m^3.

d. **False** – although '10^5 Pa' is equal to 1 atmosphere, the correct SI denotation is 100 kPa.

e. **False** – it should be '100 km s^{-1}'. The SI convention states that indicial notation – 'km s^{-1}' – should be used rather than solidus notation – 'km/s'.

7   Answers

a. **True.**

b. **False** – it, like the steradian, is a supplementary unit, not a base unit.

c. **False** – lumen is a derived unit.

d. **False** – coulomb is a derived unit.

e. **False** – farad is a derived unit.

8   Answers

a. True.
b. False – the electron-volt (eV) is not an SI unit.
c. False – the angstrom is not an SI unit.
d. False – 'centimetre water' is not an SI unit.
e. True – the radian is the measure of plane angle and the steradian of solid angle. Note: the two supplementary units are radian and steradian.

9   Answers

a. False – it is a derived SI unit.
b. True.
c. False – it is a derived SI unit.
d. True – the eV is a unit of energy. It is the energy gained by a single electron when acted on by an electric field and so accelerated through a potential of 1 V. 1 electron-volt = 1.602×10^{-19} J.
e. True.

10   Answers

a. False – the dyne is the unit of force under the cgs system and it is the force required to impart an acceleration of 1 cm s^{-1} s^{-1} to a mass of 1 g.
b. False – the cgs unit of *kinematic* viscosity. Kinematic viscosity is the ratio of the (dynamic) viscosity of a fluid (measured in poise) to its density (in grams per cubic centimetre).
c. True – henry is the SI unit of inductance.
d. False – the poise is the cgs unit of dynamic viscosity and is equal to 10^{-1} N s m^{-2} (i.e. pascal seconds).
e. True – SI unit of electrical conductance.

11   Answers

a. True – the SI unit of electrical capacitance.
b. False – lumens $\times$ seconds = talbot, which is a (non-SI) unit of light 'quantity'; cf. amperes $\times$ seconds = coulombs; watts $\times$ seconds = joules.
c. True – unit of magnetic flux density. 1 T = 10 000 gauss. Earth's magnetic flux density = 0.6 gauss.
d. True – the becquerel is the unit of radioactivity; 1 Bq is 1 nuclear disintegration s^{-1}. The previous (non-SI) unit was the curie, and 1 curie = 3.7×10^{10} Bq. Therefore, 1 curie = 37 GBq (gigabecquerel).
e. True – gray; SI unit of absorbed dose.

12   Answers

a. False – the calorie is not an SI unit; the corresponding SI unit is the joule and it is not a base unit either.
b. True – the SI unit of intensity of illumination, a base quantity.
c. False – the corresponding SI unit is the kelvin.
d. False – the corresponding unit is 10×10^{-3} m.
e. False – the coulomb is an SI unit, but it is a derived unit.

13 Answers

a. False – although the metre was first defined (in 1791) by reference to the earth's circumference it was not so defined in the SI nomenclature.

b. True – this was first introduced in 1793 and became the SI definition in 1958.

c. False – the kilometre is determined by reference to the metre and not vice versa.

d. True – this definition replaced the platinum–iridium bar definition in 1967.

e. False – the reference ought to be to the speed of light in a *vacuum*, and as such is the current definition of the metre, having replaced the krypton definition in 1983; see **2c**.

14 Answers

a. False – it is a base *unit*. The corresponding *quantity* is 'amount of substance'.

b. True.

c. False – it should be '6.02×10^{23}'; it is 10^{26} for a kilomole.

d. False – only if the solute is undissociated.

e. True – the equation is $PV = nRT$, where n refers to the number of moles.

15 Answers

a. False – it should be 101.325 kN m^{-2} or 101 325 N m^{-2}.

b. True – 1 mmHg = 1.0000001 torr.

c. False – greater by the ambient pressure, which may not necessarily be 'one standard atmosphere'.

d. True – 1 N m^{-2} is 1 Pa; 1 mmHg = 1/7.5 kPa, which is 133.3 Pa.

e. False – 10 cmH$_2$O pressure = 1 kPa. Therefore, 1 cmH$_2$O pressure = 1/10th of a kilopascal, i.e. 100 Pa.

16 Answers

a. True – 760 mmHg.

b. True.

c. False – 1 000 000 dynes cm^{-2}.

d. False – 100 kPa.

e. True.

17 Answers

a. True.

b. True.

c. True.

d. True.

e. False – it is 1 calorie, which is equal to 4.186 J.

18 Answers

a. **True** – surface tension may also be expressed in joules per square metre.

b. **True** – 1 A: the current that flows in a straight wire of infinite length if an equal current in a similar wire placed 1 m away in a vacuum produces a mutual force of 2×10^{-7} N m^{-1}.

c. **False** – electromagnetic field strength is expressed in 'volts per metre'.

d. **False** – pressure is newtons per square metre.

e. **False** – stress is a form of 'pressure' and is therefore measured in newtons per square metre.

19 Answers

a. **True.**

b. **True.**

c. **False** – strain is a ratio and therefore dimensionless.

d. **False** – surface tension is expressed in newtons per metre or joules per square metre; see **18a**.

e. **False** – newtons per unit mass. Gravitational field strength is the same as acceleration due to gravity. It is the force per unit mass, at a point in a field, acting on a mass placed at that point.

20 Answers

a. **True** – exact equivalents.

b. **True** – although formerly defined as the volume of 1 kg of pure water at 4 °C, under the metric system the litre is regarded as a special name for the cubic decimetre.

c. **True** – exact equivalents.

d. **True** – see **15b**.

e. **True** – exact equivalents because 1 N m^{-2} is the definition of the pascal.

21 Answers

a. **True.**

b. **True** – because volts × amperes = watts.

c. **True.**

d. **True.**

e. **False** – joules = watt seconds.

22 Answers

a. **False** – when using the mercury sphygmomanometer in practice its zero mark is used as the lower reference point. However, what should be the correct 'zero reference point' is the level of mercury in the reservoir, which is invisible and varies with inflation of the arm cuff. To compensate for this error the scales on the column are progressively shortened, although this is not easily discernible with the naked eye. Therefore the markings on a mercury sphygmomanometer scale are not exactly equidistant.

b. **True.**

c. **True.**

d. **False.**

e. **True.**

23 **Answers**

a. **True.**
b. **True.**
c. **False** – natural logarithms are Napierian logarithms, after John Napier (1550–1617), the Scottish mathematician. Briggsian logarithms, also known as common logarithms, are logarithms to the base 10 and were devised by Henry Briggs (1561–1630) of Oxford.
d. **False** – critical damping: a system is said to be critically damped when it reaches its equilibrium position as quickly as possible without overshooting. It has a damping factor of 1.0. Optimal damping: when the damping is c. 64% of critical, the system shows maximal speed of response with minimal overshoot and is said to be optimally damped.
e. **False.**

24 **Answers**

a. **True.**
b. **True** – although it is non-SI in nature.
c. **True** – joules per square metre is the same as newtons per metre.
d. **True** – watt seconds = joules; see **21e**.
e. **False.**

Note: surface tension is a force per unit length (which is the same as energy per unit area) acting in the surface of a liquid.

25 **Answers**

a. **False** – same as a first-order process.
b. **True** – this is the essential definition of an exponential process.
c. **True.**
d. **False** – is near complete in 4 time constants.
e. **False** – $t_{1/2}$ = 69.3% of its time constant.

26 **Answers**

a. **True.**
b. **True.**
c. **False** – the relationship is linear. This is Charles' Law.
d. **True** – it is an accelerating growth exponential.
e. **False** – the relationship is linear. This is Henry's Law.

27 **Answers**

a. **True.**
b. **False** – it is a rectangular hyperbola.
c. **False** – it is a near hyperbola.
d. **True.**
e. **False.**

28 Answers

a. **True.**
b. **False** – it is linear. This is Gay-Lussac's Law.
c. **True.**
d. **True.**
e. **True.**

Note: hysteresis is the lagging of a physical effect on a body behind its cause – *hysterein* (Gk) is 'to come late'.

29 Answers

a. **False** – laser light is collimated (see **53e**) and therefore does not obey the inverse square law.
b. **True** – this is in effect Coulomb's Law.
c. **True** – this is Graham's Law: $D \propto \dfrac{1}{\sqrt{MW}}$, which is the same as $D^2 \propto \dfrac{1}{MW}$, which is the same as $MW \propto \dfrac{1}{D^2}$.
d. **False** – energy content $\propto$ amplitude^2.
e. **False** – the relationship is inverse, not 'inverse square', but it would be true for the radius.

30 Answers

a. **True.**
b. **False** – it is a decelerating growth exponential.
c. **True.**
d. **True.**
e. **False.**

Note: wherever there is a simple inverse relationship between two quantities, i.e. $A \propto \dfrac{1}{B}$, their graphical representation takes the form of a rectangular hyperbola.

31 Answers

a. **True.**
b. **True.**
c. **True.**
d. **True.**
e. **False.**

32 Answers

a. **True** – energy $\propto$ amplitude^2.
b. **True** – $\dot{Q} \propto \sqrt{P}$; therefore $P \propto \dot{Q}^2$.
c. **True** – $\dot{Q} \propto r^4$; therefore $\dot{Q} \propto$ cross-sectional area^2.
d. **False** – energy of EMRs $\propto T^4$.
e. **True** – absorption $\propto f^2$.

33 Answers

a. True – $\omega \propto B_o$; therefore $\omega = \gamma B_o$, where γ is the gyromagnetic ratio.
b. False – the relationship is inverse; the lower the Michaelis constant, the greater the affinity.
c. False – the relationship is inverse.
d. False – diamagnetism is independent of temperature.
e. True.

34 Answers

a. True – this is Henry's Law.
b. False – it is a direct relationship but it is not linear; it is an accelerating growth exponential.
c. True – in accordance with the equation $PV = nRT$.
d. False – it is an accelerating growth exponential.
e. True – inverse relationship; the higher the frequency, the poorer the penetration.

35 Answers

a. True.
b. True.
c. True.
d. False – it is an inverse relationship; the viscosity increases with decreasing flow rate. A thixotropic fluid by definition is one whose viscosity varies inversely with its velocity.
e. False – it shows a decelerating exponential decay.

36 Answers

a. True.
b. False – it is a decelerating growth exponential.
c. True.
d. False – it is a parabola.
e. True.

37 Answers

a. True.
b. True – the variation is still sinusoidal although the frequency has vastly increased.
c. True – laser light is still a form of EMRs and therefore is propagated as a (sine) wave.
d. False.
e. True.

38 Answers

a. False.
b. False.
c. False – osmolality is osmoles of solute per *kilogram* of water, and the mass of a substance is unaffected by temperature.
d. True – the viscosity of a liquid decreases with an increase in temperature.
e. True – the latent heat of vaporization of a fluid decreases with increasing temperature.

39 Answers

a. True.

b. False – SVP is temperature dependent, not pressure dependent.

c. False – the rate of decay of a radionuclide is independent of pressure.

d. True – the viscosity of a gas increases with increasing pressure.

e. True – because the latent heat of vaporization varies with the boiling point which in turn varies with ambient pressure.

40 Answers

a. True – an ampere is 'coulomb per second'.

b. True – a watt is 'joule per second'.

c. True – lux = lumens per square metre, but 'lumen' is a rating, i.e the luminous flux – flow of light energy per unit time – per unit solid angle (steradian) from a source of 1 cd.

d. False – tesla is an 'intensity' unit; it is 'weber per square metre'.

e. True – the becquerel is the unit of radioactivity; 1 Bq is 1 nuclear disintegration s^{-1}.

41 Answers

a. False – it is the tesla that is the 'intensity' unit; see **40d**.

b. True – see **40c**.

c. False – see **40c** above.

d. False.

e. True – pascal is the unit of pressure, and 'pressure' is force/area.

42 Answers

a. True – atomic number is the number of protons in an atom; it has no units.

b. True – as the term 'relative' suggest, it is the ratio of the average mass per atom of an element to 1/12th of the mass of a carbon-12 atom. It is the same as 'atomic weight'.

c. True – it is the nucleon number, i.e. the total number of neutrons and protons in the nucleus of an atom.

d. False – 1 atomic mass unit is the same as 1 dalton.

e. True – see **b**.

43 Answers

a. False – stress is 'force per unit area', so it has the same units as 'pressure'.

b. True – 'strain' is a ratio, change in length/area/volume per unit length/area/volume.

c. False – it is the amount of a solute that passes through unit surface area (e.g. of a capillary) per unit time per unit distance (of capillary wall thickness) and is expressed in moles per square centimetre per second per centimetre thickness, i.e. moles per centimetre per second.

d. True – partition coefficient is the ratio, at equilibrium, in which an agent distributes itself between two compartments of equal volume separated by a membrane which is permeant to the agent.

e. True – also known as 'degree of substitution'. It is the ratio of substituted glucose units (i.e. those substituted with hydroxyethyl groups) to the total number of glucose molecules in hydroxyethyl starches (HESs).

44 Answers

a. False – the combining power of haemoglobin with oxygen; therefore its units are millilitres of oxygen per gram of haemoglobin.

b. False – Michaelis constant (K_m) relates to enzyme activity. It is the concentration of a substrate (moles per litre) required in order for an enzyme to act at half its maximum velocity (V_{max}), and is the measure of the affinity of an enzyme for its substrate.

c. False – Faraday constant: quantity of charge (coulombs) required to liberate one mole of monovalent (i.e. singly charged) ions in electrolysis; units: coulombs per equivalent.

d. False – Stefan constant: the constant of proportionality in the Stefan–Boltzmann equation, relating to Stefan's Law which states that the total energy radiated per unit area of a black body radiator is proportional to the fourth power of its Kelvin temperature: $E \propto T^4$. Therefore $E = \sigma T^4$, σ being the Stefan constant, whose units are: joules per second per square metre per kelvin.

e. False – also known, incorrectly, as Avogadro's number, Avogadro's constant is the number of entities – atoms or molecules – in 1 mol of substance and has the value 6.02×10^{23} mol^{-1}.

Note: as a general rule, eponymous constants (i.e. those named after persons) possess dimensions.

45 **Answers**

a. **True** – dibucaine number: percentage inhibition of the enzyme pseudocholinesterase by a 10^{-5} molar concentrate of cinchocaine (dibucaine).

b. **True** – Reynolds number = $\dfrac{v\rho d}{\eta}$, because the units of v, ρ and d of the numerator cancel out those of η of the denominator.

c. **True** – coordination number: the number of groups, molecules, atoms or ions surrounding a given atom or ion in a complex or crystal. For instance, the ferrous iron atom in the haemoglobin molecule has a coordination number of 6. Four are bonded each to a nitrogen atom of the four pyrrole rings, the fifth to an imidazole ring of a histidine residue of the α globin chain, and the sixth site is the one that combines with oxygen.

d. **False** – also known as Loschmidt's constant: the number of particles in a unit volume of an ideal gas – 2.68×10^{25} m^{-3} (cf. Avogadro's constant).

e. **False** – the former name for Avogadro's constant; see **44e**.

46 **Answers**

a. **False** – acoustic impedance: the opposition of a medium to the flow of sound waves (cf. electrical impedance). The acoustic impedance Z is equal to ρc, where ρ is the density of the medium and c is the speed of sound in it. Its units are therefore kilograms per metre^2 per second.

b. **False** – diffusion constant (also known as diffusion coefficient and diffusivity): the mass of a substance which, in diffusing from one region to another, passes through each unit of cross-sectional area per unit time when the volume-concentration gradient is unity.

c. **True** – also known as relative density, it is the ratio of the density of a substance to that of a designated reference substance, usually water.

d. **True** – dielectric constant (also known as relative permittivity) is the ratio of the absolute permittivity of the dielectric of a capacitor to the permittivity of free space. Therefore it is dimensionless.

e. **False** – The universal gas constant R is equal to PV divided by nT; its units therefore are joules per mole per kelvin.

a. **True** – fluoride number; percentage inhibition of pseudocholinesterase. Used as a test for atypical pseudocholinesterase.

b. **False** – the Quetelet index is the same as the body mass index and therefore has the units kilograms per metre^2. It is named after Lambert Adolphe Jacques Quetelet (1796–1874), the Belgian astronomer and statistician.

c. **True** – ratio of actual particles of solute present in a solution to the number of undissociated solute particles, and which therefore helps determine the true osmolarity of the solution.

d. **True** – the percentage by which the amplitude of each oscillation in a system decreases in relation to the amplitude of its preceding oscillation.

e. **False** – the gyromagnetic ratio γ is the ratio of the angular moment of an atomic system (ω) in radians per second to its magnetic moment (B_o) in tesla: $\gamma = \dfrac{\omega}{B_0}$. It is a factor relevant in the behaviour of protons in a magnetic field during magnetic resonance imaging.

48   **Answers**

a. **False** – the 'dalton' is the same as one atomic mass unit and is 1/12th of the mass of an atom of the isotope carbon-12 and is equal to 1.66033×10^{-27} kg.

b. **False** – normality of a solution is expressed in gram equivalents per litre of solution.

c. **False** – permeability is the measure of the ease with which a material is magnetized, i.e. a measure of the magnetic flux set up in a substance when a magnetic field is applied. It is therefore the ratio of the flux density B and the magnetic field strength H producing it and is designated by μ, i.e. $\mu = \dfrac{B}{H}$ henrys per metre. The permeability of free space (or magnetic constant) is that of a vacuum and is given the symbol μ_o of value $4\pi \times 10^{-7}$ H m^{-1}.

d. **False** – permittivity is a measure of the ability of a material to store electrical energy and is designated by e. It relates to the electric flux developed (as measured by the flux density, D, whose units are coulombs per metre) by a given electric field strength, E, (whose units are volts per metre). Therefore, $e = \dfrac{D}{E}$ farads per metre. The permittivity of free space (or electric constant) is that of a vacuum and is designated by e_o of value 8.854×10^{-12} F m^{-1}.

e. **False** – the mole is the SI unit of amount of substance.

49 Answers

a. True.

b. False – *Luminance* is a measure of the luminous intensity of a surface in a given direction per unit of projected area. It refers to the effectiveness of a given light on the eye, regardless of its origin, and is a physical measure of brightness. Its unit is candela per square metre ($cd\,m^{-2}$). *Illuminance* indicates the luminous power density incident on a surface such as a desk top surface or a surgical operation site. It is expressed in lumens per square metre ($lm\,m^{-2}$) or lux (lx) where 1 lx is 1 $lm\,m^{-2}$.

c. False – dynamic viscosity: newton seconds per metre^2 or pascal seconds; the units of kinematic viscosity (ratio of the dynamic viscosity of a liquid to its density) are metre^2 per second.

d. True – the unit is the ohm.

e. True – the unit is the joule (and the calorie).

50 Answers

a. False – stokes: kinematic viscosity; poise: dynamic viscosity.

b. True – the rate of disintegration of a radioactive substance; 1 Bq = 1 disintegration s^{-1}; 1 curie = $3.7 \times 10^{10}\,s^{-1}$. The becquerel is an SI unit, the curie, the former (non-SI) unit.

c. False – the henry is the unit of inductance; the inductance of a closed circuit in which an EMF of 1 V is produced when the electric current in the circuit varies uniformly at a rate of 1 A s^{-1}. The weber is the unit of magnetic flux; the flux that, when linking a circuit of one turn, produces in it an EMF of 1 V as it is reduced to 0 at a uniform rate in 1 s.

d. True – units of magnetic flux density; 1 T = 10 000 gauss.

e. False – the coulomb is the unit of electrical charge; the joule is the unit of energy.

51 Answers

a. True – unit of absorbed dose; 1 rad = 10^{-2} Gy.

b. True – units of electrical conductance; 1 siemens = 1 mho.

c. True – they both are units of force; 1 N = 10^5 dynes.

d. True – both are pressure units.

e. True – units of (radiation) dose equivalent, the siemens is the SI unit and the rem the former (non-SI) unit.

52   Answers

a. True – the weber is the SI unit of magnetic flux; the maxwell is the cgs unit of magnetic flux. I maxwell = 10^{-8} Wb.

b. False – electron-volt (eV) is a unit of energy equal to that required to move an electron through a potential difference of I V and is equal to 1.602×10^{-19} J.

c. True – the erg is the cgs unit of energy and is the work done when a force of I dyne acts through a distance of I cm; I erg = 10^{-7} J.

d. False – although both are units for measuring light energy, the lumen is a rating. It is the rate of flow of luminous energy from a light source. The talbot is the quantity of light energy that has flowed from a light source and therefore: lumens $\times$ seconds = talbots (cf. watts $\times$ seconds = joules; amperes $\times$ seconds = coulombs).

e. True – the 'dalton' is the same as one atomic mass unit and is 1/12th of the mass of an atom of the isotope carbon-12 and is equal to 1.66033×10^{-27} kg.

53   Answers

a. True.

b. True – a medium is isotropic if its physical properties are independent of direction.

c. True.

d. True.

e. False – if a beam of light is collimated (as is laser light) it does not diverge with propagation and therefore cannot obey the inverse square law.

54   Answers

a. True – converts heat energy into electrical energy.

b. True – converts electrical energy into light energy.

c. True – converts electrical energy into sound energy and vice versa.

d. False – simply changes the voltage from higher to lower.

e. False – simply adjusts the frequency of the light radiations.

55   Answers

a. True – because kinetic energy = $\frac{1}{2} mv^2$.

b. False – see **a** above.

c. True.

d. False – is increased.

e. False – the potential energy increases at the expense of the object's kinetic energy.

56   Answers

a. True – although some are capable of paramagnetism and others of ferromagnetism.

b. True – provided they are at a temperature above 0 K.

c. False – helium remains liquid at 4 K and therefore is used as a supercoolant in the MRI scanner.

d. True.

e. False – almost all; a small amount is absorbed as disaccharides.

57   Answers

a. **True** −140 000 Hz.
b. **True** – c. 50 000 Hz.
c. **False** – the frequency is c. 2.4 GHz.
d. **False** – the frequency is in the terahertz (i.e. 10^3 gigahertz) range.
e. **True** – 10^5 Hz range.

58   Answers

a. **False** – it varies inversely with temperature; the viscosity of a gas varies directly with temperature.
b. **False** – there is no relationship between the density and the viscosity of a liquid. For example, water (density: 1 g ml^{-1}) is denser than di-ethyl ether (0.736 g ml^{-1}) but has a much lower viscosity (at 20 °C): water: 1 mPa s; ether: 2.34 mPa s).
c. **True** – flow rates of fluids have an inverse relation with their viscosities, as indicated by the Hagen–Poiseuille equation: $\dot{Q} \propto \frac{1}{\eta}$.
d. **True** – Reynolds number = $\frac{v\rho d}{\eta}$, where v = velocity of fluid flow; ρ = density of fluid; d = diameter of the tube; and η = viscosity of the fluid.
e. **False** – the units are pascal seconds (i.e. newton seconds per metre^2).

59   Answers

a. **False** – in laminar flow viscosity is the determining factor. Density is a factor in turbulent flow.
b. **True** – kinematic viscosity is dynamic viscosity divided by density.
c. **False** – flow in the lower regions of anaesthetic machine flowmeter tubes is tubular and laminar and is therefore influenced by the gas's viscosity. In the upper regions it is orificial and turbulent and therefore affected by the agent's density.
d. **True** – heat capacity is the amount of heat required to raise the temperature of a known *volume* of substance by 1 °C. If the substance has been quantified in terms of mass then its density is a material factor in determining its volume.
e. **True** – because the flow is orificial and therefore turbulent, and in turbulent flow density is a material factor.

60   Answers

a. **True** – in the lower part of the tube (low flows) viscosity is the relevant property, in the higher part (higher flows) it is density.
b. **False** – density has no part in laminar flow.
c. **True** – Reynolds number = $\frac{v\rho d}{\eta}$.
d. **True** – because kinematic viscosity = dynamic viscosity/density.
e. **False** – only density plays a part.

61   Answers

a. True.
b. True.
c. True.
d. False – it is the presence of van der Waals forces that makes gases non-ideal.
e. False – it is not a definitional attribute of an ideal gas that it shall have a critical temperature below 0 °C.

62   Answers

a. False – an ideal gas conforms in its behaviour to the Ideal Gas equation: $PV = nRT$; it is a non-ideal gas that conforms to van der Waals equation of state: $(p + a/V^2)(V - b) = RT$.
b. True – an ideal gas has no means of storing energy except as translational kinetic energy. It is this inability to store energy that makes the collisions between the molecules themselves and those between the molecules and the walls of their container perfectly elastic.
c. True – because kinetic energy is solely temperature dependent.
d. False – the latent heat of vaporization of a gas, be it ideal or non-ideal, decreases with increasing temperature.
e. False.

63   Answers

a. True – the ideal gas equation states that $PV = nRT$. For an oxygen cylinder V (the internal volume of the cylinder) is constant. R and T are constants. Therefore $P \propto n$; i.e. the pressure (as indicated on the Bourdon gauge) is a function of the number of moles of gas in the cylinder.
b. False – it is Boyle's Law. $P_1 V_1 = P_2 V_2$. For instance, a size E oxygen cylinder will give 680 L of oxygen (at a pressure of 1 atmosphere). If the internal volume of the cylinder is y litres, then, $P_1 V_1$ being equal to $P_2 V_2$, 137 (pressure of a full cylinder) $\times y$ (internal volume) = $(680 + y) \times 1$, y being the volume of gas remaining in the cylinder (at 1 bar). Therefore, $(680 + y) \times 1 = 137 \times y$, and $y = 680/136 = 5$. A similar calculation can be applied to an air cylinder or indeed any cylinder whose contents are solely gaseous.
c. False – the relationship between shear rate and shear stress is indicated by the viscosity, which is a factor in the Hagen–Poiseuille equation. However, this only applies to laminar flow, not to turbulent flow.
d. True – Gay-Lussac's Law states that the pressure of a fixed mass of gas at constant volume is proportional to its temperature. Therefore the pressure of the saturated vapour of desflurane at 39 °C (the temperature of the vaporizing chamber of the desflurane vaporizer) is above atmospheric and is in fact about 2 bar.
e. False – it is Gay-Lussac's Law for the same reason as in the case of the desflurane vaporizer; see **63d**.

64   Answer

a. True – Raoult's Law: the partial vapour pressure of a solvent is proportional to its mole fraction. If p is the vapour pressure of a solvent (with a substance in solution in it) and X the mole fraction of solvent (number of moles of solvent as a fraction of the total number of moles) then $p = p_oX$, where p_o is the vapour pressure of the pure solvent (cf. Dalton's Law of partial pressures).

b. True.

c. True – Raoult's Law only holds for dilute solutions. But some mixtures of liquids obey it over a wider range of concentrations, and these are known as perfect solutions.

d. True – an azeotrope is a liquid mixture that is characterized by a constant minimum or maximum boiling point, which is lower or higher than that of any of its components, and that distils without any change in composition. Azeotropes in their behaviour show a large deviation from an ideal mixture.

e. True.

65   Answers

a. True – Gay-Lussac's Law: the pressure of a fixed mass of gas of constant volume is proportional to its Kelvin temperature. Therefore if the temperature is raised the pressure will increase proportionately. The temperature of the vaporizing chamber is 39 °C (312 K) and therefore the (vapour) pressure is higher c. 1500 mmHg.

b. True – an autoclave usually operates at a temperature of c.134 °C, at which temperature the steam is at a pressure of about 1.39 bar.

c. True – a Bourdon gauge can be used to detect pressure change in relation to temperature change in a fixed mass of gas at constant volume.

d. False – it is the Bernoulli phenomenon and Venturi effect that apply here.

e. False.

66   Answers

a. True.

b. True.

c. False – it is at its 'Boyle temperature' that a gas most closely approximates to an ideal gas.

d. True.

e. False.

67   Answers

a. True.

b. False – $\dot{Q} \propto P$.

c. False – the viscosity is constant in a Newtonian fluid because by definition such a fluid conforms to laminar flow.

d. False – density is not an operating factor in the flow of a Newtonian fluid.

e. True – because $\dot{Q} \propto r^4$, and r^4 holds the same 'proportionality' to $\dot{Q}$ in the Hagen–Poiseuille equation as does the square of the cross-sectional area.

68   Answers

a. **False.**
b. **True.**
c. **True.**
d. **False.**
e. **False.**

69   Answers

a. **True** – a polar compound is one that is either ionic (e.g. sodium chloride) or that has molecules with a large permanent dipole moment. Water belongs to the latter category because of its hydrogen bonds.
b. **False** – the H–O–H angle of water is 105 degrees.
c. **True** – dielectric constant is 80 (that for a vacuum is 1).
d. **True.**
e. **False** – absorbs infrared light.

70   Answers

a. **True.**
b. **True** – i.e. it can act both as an acid and as an alkali.
c. **True.**
d. **False** – a good solvent for aliphatic compounds.
e. **True.**

71   Answers

a. **True.**
b. **True.**
c. **True.**
d. **False.**
e. **True** – the non-Newtonian nature of blood is due to the presence of red cells *and* fibrinogen together; remove either of them and the fluid beomes near-Newtonian.

72   Answers

a. **True** – there are no 'degrees' of it; hence the absence of a degree sign (°) in its denotation.
b. **True.**
c. **True.**
d. **True.**
e. **True.**

73   Answers

a. **False** – the solubility decreases.
b. **False** – the rate of disintegration of a radionuclide is independent of temperature.
c. **True** – the relationship is that of an accelerating growth exponential.
d. **False** – the viscosity of a liquid is inversely related to its temperature.
e. **False** – the speed of light in a vacuum is a constant at $299\,792\,458$ m s^{-1}.

74   Answers

a. True – it increases with temperature.

b. False – since osmolality is the number of solute particles per *kilogram* of water and since the mass of any substance is not temperature dependent, its osmolality is unaffected by temperature. It is different for *osmolarity*, because here it is the *volume* of the solution, and not the mass of the solvent, that is material, and volume varies with temperature. If it is a polar solute in solution, then the degree of dissociation of the solute may be temperature dependent and therefore may determine the osmolality of the solution.

c. True – above a certain temperature, the *Curie* temperature, a ferromagnetic substance becomes paramagnetic.

d. False – diamagnetism is unaffected by temperature.

e. True – the higher the temperature, the higher the frequency; see **78a–c**.

75   Answers

a. True – expansion of a metal (mercury thermometer), other liquid (alcohol) or a gas (gas thermometer).

b. True – infrared thermometer.

c. True – platinum resistance thermometer.

d. True – Bourdon gauge thermometer.

e. True – if an electric current is passed across transistor junctions, the voltage developed is temperature dependent.

76   Answers

a. True – a positive temperature coefficient of expansion.

b. True – a positive temperature coefficient of expansion.

c. True – a positive temperature coefficient of electrical resistance.

d. True – a positive coefficient of potential difference.

e. False – a negative coefficient of resistance because the thermistor is made of semiconductor material, and semiconductors decrease their electrical resistance with a rise in temperature.

77   Answers

a. True – over the range of 0–100 °C the change in resistance is linear with temperature change and is c. 0.4 ohms per °C for a 100 ohm resistance element.

b. False.

c. False.

d. True.

e. True – a gas expands by equal volumes for each degree rise in temperature (Charles' Law).

Answers

a. **True** – Wien's Law of displacement: the wavelength of maximum energy emission of a black body radiator (a perfect radiator, also referred to as a 'perfect black body') is inversely related to its Kelvin temperature.

b. **True** – the Stefan–Boltzmann equation is based on the fact that for a black body radiator the rate of emission of total radiation energy is proportional to the fourth power of its Kelvin temperature, i.e. $E \propto T^4$. Therefore, $E = \sigma T^4$, where σ is the Stefan constant, whose units are joules per second per $kelvin^4$.

c. **True** – the energy of EMRs is directly proportional to the frequency of the EMRs. (Note: this is Wien's Law in a different guise). Therefore, $E \propto f$ and $E = h f$, where h is the Planck constant and has the value 6.626×10^{-34} J s.

d. **False** – Larmor frequency is relevant to the working of the MRI scanner and is the frequency of *precession* of charged particles in a magnetic field. In the case of MRI the charged particles are hydrogen protons, the magnetic field is 1–3 T, and the frequency of precession is in the radiofrequency range.

e. **False** – Soret peak has nothing to do with infrared radiations. It is the spectral absorbance maximum exhibited by cytochrome P 450 enzyme at 450 nm when reduced and complexed with carbon monoxide.

79 **Answers**

a. **True.**

b. **True** – so, the value of a given temperature displayed during a heating cycle is different from the value displayed for the same temperature during the cooling cycle.

c. **False** – thermistors generally have a much higher temperature coefficient than resistance thermometers. Therefore they can be used to detect much smaller temperature variations.

d. **False** – fast response time.

e. **True** – but this can be corrected by the use of appropriate electronic circuitry.

80 **Answers**

a. **True** – as its name suggests.

b. **True.**

c. **False** – it detects a change in potential difference.

d. **False** – it detects a change in coefficient of expansion.

e. **False** – it detects a change in gas pressure.

81   Answers

a. True – it converts heat energy into mechanical energy.

b. True – by expansion of the volume of the mercury in the device.

c. False – mercury does not have a high enough coefficient of expansion for the purpose; it only increases by about 1.8% of its volume over an increase of 100 °C; but it is used because it is very consistent in its performance.

d. True – because the volume change is very small it has to be converted into a very long, and therefore very fine, capillary column of mercury. This makes it difficult to read. Hence the need for a lens on the surface of the thermometer stem to magnify the width of the column and render it more visible.

e. True – the use of mercury in equipment and appliances used for clinical purposes has been outlawed under EC regulations.

82   Answers

a. True.

b. True – melting point 1773 °C.

c. True.

d. False – about 20 times less sensitive.

e. False – slower response time because of its high thermal capacity.

83   Answers

a. True.

b. False – less stable.

c. True – about 20 times as sensitive as the platinum resistance thermometer.

d. True – very small thermal capacity.

e. True – because of its smaller thermal capacity.

84   Answers

a. True.

b. False.

c. True.

d. True.

e. False.

Note: provided the agent in the cylinder is entirely gaseous, its amount can be determined by applying the Universal Gas equation, $PV = nRT$. V, R and T are constants and therefore $P \propto n$ (number of moles and therefore the amount of gas).

85   Answers

a. True – in other words, there is not a 'carbon trioxide' or 'carbon tetroxide'.

b. False – produced for medical use: (i) as a byproduct gas during manufacture of hydrogen; (ii) as a byproduct gas from fermentation; and (iii) as a combustion gas from burning fuel.

c. False.

d. True.

e. False – as an exothermic reaction.

Answers

a. **False** – greenhouse effect relative potencies: CO_2: 1; CH_4: 11; N_2O: 270; CFCs: 7100. The greater effect of CO_2 is due to the fact that it is released in much greater amounts than all the other greenhouse gases combined.

b. **False** – CO_2: 31.4 °C; N_2O: 36.4 °C.

c. **False.**

d. **False** – viscosity at 1 bar and 25 °C –CO_2: 0.0150 mPa s; O_2: 0.0208 mPa s.

e. **True** – CO_2: 0.03; helium: 0.0005.

87 **Answers**

a. **True** – Pasteur point: critical PO_2 value below which aerobic metabolism cannot occur in mitochondria. It is taken as being 0.15–0.3 kPa (1.4–2.3 mmHg).

b. **True** – combining power of haemoglobin (in grams) with oxygen (in millilitres).

c. **False** – Peltier effect: change in temperature that results at a junction between two dissimilar metals or semiconductors when an electric current passes through the junction.

d. **False** – Hamburger phenomenon: chloride shift from plasma into red cells following bicarbonate formation from CO_2 in venous blood.

e. **False** – Circe effect: utilization of attractive forces on an enzyme so as to lure a substrate to the enzyme's active site at which the substrate undergoes biochemical transformation of its structure. It is named after the Greek goddess, *Circe*, who is said to have lured Odysseus's men to her house and then transformed them into pigs.

88 **Answers**

a. **True** – because it has two unpaired electrons in its outer shell.

b. **True** – diradical: a radical that has two unpaired electrons at different points in the molecule so that the radical centres are independent of each other. Radical: a molecular fragment with an odd number of unshared electrons.

c. **True** – just as well, otherwise life on earth will come to a premature end!

d. **True** – hence the tendency on the part of nurses to ask doctors to write on a patient's prescription chart if they want the patient to have postoperative oxygen on the ward.

e. **True** – any gas can be analysed by mass spectrometry.

89 **Answers**

a. **False.**

b. **True** – oxygen: 0.0208; N_2O: 0.0147 at 25 °C.

c. **True** – but its partial pressure varies because the (total) atmospheric pressure of gases varies with height above sea level.

d. **False** – as two allotropes: oxygen and ozone.

e. **True** – O^{16}, O^{17} and O^{18} in the ratio 1000:3.7:20.

90 Answers

a. False – oxygen has two electrically identical atoms in covalent linkage in its molecule and therefore there is no 'polarity' between the two atoms.

b. False – only present in nature as nonradioactive isotopes; see **89e**. Unstable isotopes of oxygen – O^{14}, O^{15}, O^{19} and O^{20} – have been prepared artificially, but they all have very short half-lives and do not occur in natural oxygen.

c. True – critical pressure: the minimum pressure required to liquefy a gas at its critical temperature.

d. False.

e. True.

91 Answers

a. True – Joule–Thomson effect: adiabatic expansion, which is the process involved in the manufacture of oxygen by the fractional distillation of air.

b. True – Allis–Chalmers process: electrochemical process for preparing oxygen by ionizing oxygen in air at one electrode of a cell and then recovering the gas in its pure form at the other electrode. It is not an economical method and has been superseded by the method of fractional distillation of air.

c. False – the tendency of nitrous oxide to remain gaseous under pressure even when below its critical temperature when mixed with oxygen.

d. True – liquefaction of air, first achieved by Hampson and von Linde in 1895.

e. False – Paul Bert effect: acute oxygen poisoning of the CNS as a result of breathing 100% oxygen under hyperbaric conditions.

92 Answers

a. True.

b. True.

c. True.

d. False.

e. True.

93 Answers

a. True – see **91e**.

b. False – Cushing effect: bradycardia and hypertension as a result of acutely raised intracranial pressure.

c. True – Lorrain–Smith effect: damage to pulmonary epithelium as a result of prolonged inhalation of 100% oxygen.

d. False – Poseiro effect: decrease in arterial blood pressure during contractions of a gravid uterus, thought to be due to exacerbations of aorto-caval compression.

e. False – Fahraeus–Lindqvist effect: alignment of red blood cells as they pass through small vessels; instead of moving randomly, the red cells line up and move through the vessel 'single file', thereby minimizing the viscous resistance that would otherwise occur.

a. **True.**
b. **False** – needs to be breathed for 12–24 hours to cause substernal discomfort.
c. **True** – convulsions can occur: Paul Bert effect.
d. **True.**
e. **True** – related to the Lorrain–Smith effect; see **93c**.

95 **Answers**

a. **True.**
b. **False** – pressure is a manifestation of potential energy.
c. **True** – because the Universal Gas equation – $PV = nRT$ – is correctly applicable to it.
d. **False.**
e. **False** – 'filling ratio' does not apply to oxygen cylinders because their contents are solely gaseous.

96 **Answers**

a. **True.**
b. **True.**
c. **True.**
d. **False** – in fact it is customary to have the reserve bank of oxygen cylinders (size J) sited adjacent to the VIE.
e. **True.**

97 **Answers**

a. **False** – it is an allotrope of oxygen.
b. **False.**
c. **True.**
d. **True.**
e. **True** – CO: 100 ppm; ozone: 1 ppm. Ozone is not tolerated in industrial establishments in concentrations greater than 1 ppm whereas CO can be tolerated in strengths as high as 100 ppm.

98 **Answers**

a. **True.**
b. **False** – but it has been known to vitiate oxygen analysis by some paramagnetic analysers.
c. **True** – although it has a latent tendency to decompose into its elements, nitrous oxide is kinetically stable at room temperatures. But N_2O can decompose at 400–500 °C.
d. **False** – although hyponitrous acid decomposes easily to form nitrous oxide and water: $H_2N_2O_2 \rightarrow N_2O + H_2O$, nitrous oxide does not recombine with water to form acid.
e. **False.**

99 Answers

a. False – Paul Bert effect: acute oxygen poisoning of the CNS as a result of breathing 100% oxygen under hyperbaric conditions.
b. False.
c. False.
d. True – Fink phenomenon: diffusion hypoxia.
e. True – increased alveolar concentration of N_2O (a less soluble gas) following rapid uptake of a concomitantly administered more soluble agent such as isoflurane.

100 Answers

a. True.
b. True.
c. False – in the UK CO_2 is produced from three sources: (i) as a byproduct gas from manufacture of hydrogen; (ii) as a byproduct gas from fermentation; and (iii) as a combustion gas from burning fuel.
d. False – from natural gas.
e. True.

101 Answers

a. True.
b. False – argon: 0.93%; xenon: 0.000008%.
c. True – MAC: xenon: 71; N_2O: 105.
d. True.
e. True.

102 Answers

a. True – xenon: 131.3; nitrous oxide: 44.
b. False – xenon: 71; nitrous oxide: 105.
c. False – xenon: 16.5 °C; nitrous oxide: 36.4 °C.
d. False – xenon: 0.14; nitrous oxide: 0.47.
e. False – neither undergoes biotransformation.

103 Answers

a. False – (at 20 °C and 1 bar) xenon: 5.88 g/L; nitrous oxide: 1.53 g/L.
b. True – (at 20° C and 1 bar) xenon: 0.0227 mPa s; nitrous oxide: 0.0147 mPa s.
c. True – xenon: –108 °C; nitrous oxide: –88 °C.
d. False – because nitrous oxide has a higher blood gas partition coefficient.
e. True – because nitrous oxide has a lower molecular weight: Graham's Law of diffusion.

104 Answers

a. True.
b. False – to be amenable to assay by infrared analysis a gas must have at least two dissimilar atoms in its molecule.
c. True – (at 20 °C and 1 bar) xenon: 5.887 g/L; air 1.00 g/L.
d. False – (at 20 °C and 1 bar) xenon: 0.0227 mPa s; oxygen: 0.0196 mPa s.
e. False.

105 Answers

a. **True** – also known as the overpressure effect, the Poynting effect (after John Henry Poynting [1852–1914], the British physicist), is the conversion of pressurized liquid nitrous oxide into nitrous oxide vapour by mixing it with gaseous oxygen at high pressure.

b. **True.**

c. **True.**

d. **False** – Fink phenomenon (after Raymond Fink, Seattle anaesthesiologist): diffusion hypoxia resulting at the end of a N_2O-containing general anaesthetic, when the patient is allowed to breathe room air.

e. **False.**

106 Answers

a. **False** – from natural gas.

b. **True** – hence its use as a supercoolant in the MRI scanner.

c. **False** – argon: 0.93%; helium: 0.0005%.

d. **False** – viscosity (at 1 bar and 20 °C): helium: 0.0198 mPa s; nitrogen: 0.0179 mPa s.

e. **False** – primarily to avoid the effect of narcosis with hyperbaric nitrogen.

107 Answers

a. **True** – because of its relative insolubility in blood.

b. **True** – to maintain 'population inversion' of carbon dioxide, the lasing medium.

c. **False.**

d. **True** – as a supercryogen to reduce energy costs in producing the magnetic field of the electromagnetic radiation.

e. **False** – it is carbon monoxide that is used for this purpose.

108 Answers

a. **True.**

b. **True.**

c. **True.**

d. **True** – but this effect is slight and of no practical importance.

e. **False.**

109 Answers

a. **False.**

b. **True.**

c. **False.**

d. **False.**

e. **True.**

110 Answers

a. **False.**

b. **False.**

c. **False.**

d. **False.**

e. **True.**

111 Answers

a. **True.**
b. **False** – about 54 bar at room temperature.
c. **True.**
d. **True.**
e. **True.**

112 Answers

a. **False.**
b. **True.**
c. **True.**
d. **False.**
e. **False.**

113 Answers

a. **True** – CO: 100 ppm; ozone: 1 ppm; ozone is not tolerated in industrial establishments in concentrations greater than 1 ppm, whereas CO can be tolerated in strengths as high as 100 ppm.
b. **True** – H_2S: 100 ppm; ozone: 1 ppm.
c. **True** – HCN: 10 ppm; ozone: 1 ppm.
d. **True** – NO_2: 25–100 ppm; ozone: 1 ppm.
e. **True** – SO_2: 25–50 ppm; ozone: 1 ppm.

114 Answers

a. **False.**
b. **False.**
c. **False.**
d. **True.**
e. **True.**

Note: the answers to this MCQ ought to be easy provided you bear Graham's Law in mind and know the molecular weights of the agents. Graham's Law: the rate of diffusion of a gas down its concentration gradient is inversely proportional to the square root

of its molecular weight: $D \propto \dfrac{1}{\sqrt{MW}}$.

Molecular weights:
N_2O: 44; O_2: 32; CO_2: 44; NO: 28; diethyl ether: 74; xenon: 131.

115 Answers

a. **True.**
b. **False.**
c. **False.**
d. **True.**
e. **True.**

a. **False** – named after Henry Edmund Gaskin Boyle (1875–1941) anaesthetist at St Bartholomew's Hospital. Robert Boyle (of Boyle's Law fame) (1627–1691) was a natural philosopher at Oxford University and was a Founder member of the Royal Society.

b. **False** – still needs antistatic precautions so as to prevent the bobbins sticking inside the rotameter flow tubes. This is provided by lining the inside walls of the flowmeter tubes with aluminium oxide or tin oxide.

c. **False** – the flow pressure up the flowtubes is about one-third of an atmosphere (c. 35 kPa).

d. **False** – no pressure regulators are necessary because the pipeline supply is already at about 4 bar pressure.

e. **False** – no longer necessary as flammable anaesthetic agents are no longer in use.

117 Answers

a. **True.**

b. **True.**

c. **False.**

d. **False** – air if provided should not to be cut off.

e. **False.**

118 Answers

a. **False** – the oxygen flowmeter may yet be positioned at the left-hand end, but the agent itself shall join the common gas pathway downstream of the other gases.

b. **True.**

c. **True.**

d. **False** – while a visual alarm may be incorporated, it is not mandatory under ISO regulations.

e. **False.**

119 Answers

a. **False** – according to ISO regulations the oxygen cut-off warning device shall be *activated by oxygen and oxygen alone*.

b. **True** – has a 'reservoir' of about 200 ml of oxygen at 4 bar to activate the whistle.

c. **False** – air should not be cut off.

d. **False** – minimum of 7 s.

e. **True** – i.e. sound intensity of ordinary sitting room conversation.

120 Answers

a. **False** – upstream of the pressure regulators.

b. **True.**

c. **False** – must be made of nonflammable material so that it does not catch fire from the heat generated during adiabatic compression that may occur at the cylinder–machine interface when high pressure gases impact on the Bodok seal.

d. **False** – adiabatic compression; see **c** above.

e. **True** – because mineral oil can explode with high pressure oxygen.

121 Answers

a. False – variable orifice, constant pressure differential principle.
b. True – they are of different lengths and/or bores.
c. False – accurate to within 2–4%.
d. False – deliver gases along them at a pressure of about one-third of an atmosphere (c. 33–35 kPa).
e. True – to prevent the bobbins from sticking.

122 Answers

a. False – the gas pressure of 4 bar stops at the needle valve at the bottom of the flowmeter tubes.
b. True.
c. True.
d. True.
e. False – the Manley MP 3 ventilator is driven by the gases that flow down the 'back bar', which are at a pressure of about one-third atmosphere.

123 Answers

a. True.
b. False – at 35–40 L min^{-1}.
c. False – to match the patient's peak inspiratory flow rate.
d. False – it should be operable only by keeping its control button held down manually.
e. False – but it will reduce the flow rate up the O_2 flowmeter tube.

124 Answers

a. True.
b. True.
c. True.
d. False.
e. False.

125 Answers

a. False – size F oxygen cylinders (i) do not have pin index outlets and (ii) are too tall for attaching to an anaesthetic machine.
b. True – because their contents are partly liquid, and so must CO_2 and cyclopropane cylinders.
c. True – C, D or E, but size D is the most common.
d. False – its contents are partly liquid and therefore a pressure gauge gives no accurate indication of the amount of agent in the cylinder.
e. False – cyclopropane does not, because a 'full' cylinder is at a pressure of only about 5–7 bar.

126 Answers

a. **True** – 'plenum' means 'full', i.e. 'full' of air.
b. **False** – temperature compensation and plenum provision are two different features satisfying two different purposes.
c. **True.**
d. **False** – the 'Boyle bottle', which pre-dates TEC vaporizers, is a plenum vaporizer.
e. **False** – but as a TEC vaporizer it invariably is, so as to provide a large 'heatsink'.

127 Answers

a. **True.**
b. **False.**
c. **True.**
d. **True.**
e. **False.**

Note: the desflurane and Halox vaporizers are based on the (Lucien Morris) 'copper kettle' principle.

128 Answers

a. **True** – the partial pressure of an anaesthetic vapour is not dependent on ambient pressure, but on temperature. Therefore, if the temperature is the same, the vaporizer will deliver the agent vapour at the same pressure as at sea level. However, the total pressure of the gas mixture is lower than that at sea level and therefore the vapour will form a higher percentage of the gas mixture, i.e. a higher volumes per cent.
b. **False** – for the same reasons as **a**, i.e. provided the temperature is the same, the vaporizer will deliver the agent at the same partial pressure of the agent. But since the chamber is hyperbaric the agent vapour will form a smaller percentage (by volume) of the total gas mixture. But since the pressure is higher the density of the vapour has increased proportionately, and therefore the final mass of agent output from the vaporizer is unaltered.
c. **False** – helium-enriched carrier gas mixtures are likely to reduce the output concentration of the vaporizer.
d. **True.**
e. **False** – the output will be higher because the saturation vapour pressure of an agent increases with increasing temperature.

129 Answers

a. **False** – the Boyle bottle does not provide a means of temperature compensation, heatsink or other.
b. **False** – by means of an ether bellows, which serves the same function as the bimetallic strip of TEC vaporizers, although there is a heatsink in the form of a water chamber.
c. **False** – by means of a bimetallic strip.
d. **False** – by means of a bimetallic strip.
e. **False** – by provision of extraneous heat by electrical means.

130 Answers

a. True.
b. True.
c. True.
d. True.
e. True – the internal resistance to gas flow is about 50 cmH$_2$O pressure per 10 L per minute flow rate.

131 Answers

a. True.
b. False.
c. True – because there would be a larger 'air gap' above the fluid level for back-pressured gases to pick up more agent.
d. True.
e. True.

132 Answers

a. False – e.g. the Boyle bottle is a plenum vaporizer but not a TEC vaporizer, while the EMO (Epstein–Oxford–Macintosh) is a TEC vaporizer but is normally used as a draw-over vaporizer.
b. True.
c. False – by means of a bimetallic strip.
d. True.
e. False – the internal resistance is too high, up to 50 cmH$_2$O pressure at a flow rate of c. 10 L min^{-1}.

133 Answers

a. True.
b. False – primarily by the performance of the bimetallic strip.
c. True.
d. False – some vaporizers, such as the Sevoflurane vaporizer, have the control dial face in the vertical plane.
e. True – the Goldman (draw-over) vaporizer can be used as a plenum vaporizer, but the TEC Mark 4 (plenum vaporizer) cannot be used as a draw-over vaporizer.

134 Answers

a. False – Mark 6.
b. True.
c. False – it can be filled during its warm-up cycle and indeed even when in use.
d. True – because desflurane has a higher MAC and therefore more agent is required for the same gas flow rate. Its capacity is about 425 ml; Mark 4 TEC vaporizers have a capacity of about 350 ml.
e. True – but needs mains electricity to maintain the chamber temperature at 39 °C.

135   Answers

a. **False** – because the Manley MP 3 ventilator is a 'minute volume divider' the ventilation rate is equal to the minute volume (fresh gas flow rate) divided by the tidal volume. Change the tidal volume and the ventilation rate changes inversely with it.

b. **True** – because the tidal volume and ventilation rate are independently settable and neither is dependent on the fresh gas flow rate.

c. **True** – by use of a Newton valve, as when it is used for paediatric ventilation.

d. **False** –the Pneupac is based on the Bernoulli phenomenon and Venturi effect and therefore air is entrained by means of a supply of pressurized oxygen. Of course, if pressurized air is used instead of oxygen then the machine can deliver air alone. But this will necessitate re-configuring of the connections, which is not a practical proposition.

e. **True** –because it is capable of maintaining a very high pressure differential (between ventilator bellows and the patient's alveoli) during the inspiratory phase. In practice, the delivered tidal volume is limited by (i) the pre-set inspiratory time and (ii) the end-inspiratory pressure, which when it has reached a certain maximum safe limit will provide for gas escape through a safety valve, so as to prevent barotrauma to the lungs.

136   Answers

a. **False** – but the only constant pressure generator ventilator in common use, the Manley MP 3, is a minute volume divider.

b. **False** – shows a negative decelerating exponential change.

c. **False** – since the delivery of gases during inspiration is exponential, it will come to an end in 4 time constants and further prolongation of the inspiratory phase will not by itself increase the tidal volume delivered.

d. **False** – because it is a pressure generator, any fall in the patient's lung compliance will restrict the tidal volume delivered.

e. **False** – it is exemplified by the Manley MP 3 ventilator. The Penlon AV 900 ventilator is a constant flow generator ventilator.

137   Answers

a. **True.**

b. **True.**

c. **False.**

d. **True.**

e. **False** – by definition a 'static' measurement can only apply when there is no movement of gas in the system.

138   Answers

a. **True.**

b. **False.**

c. **True.**

d. **True.**

e. **True.**

139 Answers

a. **True.**
b. **True.**
c. **True.**
d. **False.**
e. **True** – more recently introduced light-weight cylinders, which are particularly useful for patient transfer and essential for patients during investigations in the MRI unit.

140 Answers

a. **False.**
b. **True.**
c. **False.**
d. **False.**
e. **False.**

Note: any cylinder whose contents are partly liquid must be mounted vertically during use.

141 Answers

a. **False.**
b. **True.**
c. **True.**
d. **False.**
e. **True.**

142 Answers

a. **False.**
b. **True.**
c. **False.**
d. **False** – under-reads at low volumes and over-reads at high volumes.
e. **True.**

143 Answers

a. **False** – because the contents of a 'full' CO_2 cylinder are partly liquid.
b. **True.**
c. **False** – from a circle to an ellipse with a fall in pressure.
d. **True.**
e. **True.**

144 Answers

a. **True.**
b. **True.**
c. **False.**
d. **False.**
e. **True.**

145 Answers

a. **False** – Mapleson A attachment.

b. **True** – because the source of fresh gas(es) is the anaesthetic machine (as opposed to atmospheric air) and the destination of the exhaled gases is at least partly the atmosphere.

c. **True.**

d. **False** – the parallel Lack attachment is said to be the most efficient breathing attachment for spontaneous ventilation because, of all attachments, it requires the smallest fresh gas flow rate in relation to minute volume to maintain near-normocapnia.

e. **True.**

146 Answers

a. **True** – because the attachment is a 'semi-closed' one and therefore there is no provision for air entrainment if the fresh gas flow were to fall short of the patient's minute volume. Therefore the patient will have to make up the shortfall in fresh gas flow required to match the alveolar ventilation volume by retaining some part of the exhaled tidal volume. This will lead to re-breathing and thus a rise in end-tidal CO_2.

b. **False** – if the APL valve remains 'open' during inspiration the patient may entrain air through it. This may lighten the anaesthetic but there will not necessarily be a rise in end-tidal CO_2.

c. **False.**

d. **False.**

e. **True** – if the bag is detached from the bag mount, the point of admixture of fresh gases and exhaled gases will move further 'upstream' from the APL valve site to the bag mount site. This will lead to a huge rise in apparatus dead space with a consequent rise in end-tidal CO_2.

147 Answers

a. **True.**

b. **False.**

c. **False.**

d. **True.**

e. **True.**

148 Answers

a. **False** – it is a Mapleson D.

b. **False** – outer co-axial efferent limb. The co-axial Lack attachment has an outer co-axial afferent limb.

c. **False** – more efficient.

d. **False** – predominantly exhaled gases.

e. **False** – because the apparatus dead space would be hardly changed. But if the disconnection occurred at the CGO end then there will be a massive increase in the apparatus dead space, leading to extreme hypercapnia.

Note: Other things being equal, the ET CO_2 is directly proportional to the ratio of dead space to alveolar fraction. Therefore, an increase in the dead space, be it anatomical, alveolar or apparatus dead space, will increase the ET CO_2.

149 Answers

a. **False** – Mapleson C.
b. **False** – a mixture of fresh gas and expired gas.
c. **True** – by incorporating a soda lime canister between the patient end and 'breathing' bag.
d. **False** – because it contains a spring-loaded valve as an expiratory port, and spring-loaded valves should be avoided in paediatric breathing attachments because of their high resistance to expiration.
e. **True.**

150 Answers

a. **True.**
b. **False.**
c. **False.**
d. **True.**
e. **True.**

151 Answers

a. **False** – hypercapnia will follow if the fresh gas flow is less than the alveolar ventilation volume.
b. **True.**
c. **False** – hypercapnia will follow if the fresh gas flow is less than the alveolar ventilation volume.
d. **True.**
e. **True.**

152 Answers

a. **True.**
b. **True.**
c. **True.**
d. **False.**
e. **False.**

153 Answers

a. **False** – it is an exothermic reaction.
b. **True** – the 'catalyst' is sodium hydroxide.
c. **False** – the reaction is irreversible.
d. **True** – water is necessary for the initial chemical reaction: $CO_2 + H_2O \rightarrow H_2CO_3$.
e. **True** – one molecule of water is used up (see **d** above) and two molecules are produced.

154 Answers

a. True.

b. True – it has been shown that Baralyme (which contains 4.6% potassium hydroxide) produced more CO with desflurane, enflurane and isoflurane than does soda lime (which contains only 2.5% potassium hydroxide).

c. True.

d. False.

e. True – the order of producing CO with soda lime by the various inhalational agents is: desflurane > enflurane > isoflurane >> halothane = sevoflurane.

155 Answers

a. False – acetone accumulates because it has been released by the (starving) patient.

b. True – CO is more likely to be produced by those anaesthetic agents having a CHF_2 moiety, viz desflurane, isoflurane and enflurane.

c. True – produced by halothane.

d. False – methane is released by the patient.

e. True – used to be produced if trichloroethylene were to be used with soda lime; trichloroethylene is no longer used as an anaesthetic agent.

156 Answers

a. True.

b. True – generated by sevoflurane in accordance with the Cannizzaro disproportionation reaction (named after Stanislao Cannizaro [1826–1910], the Italian chemist): a reaction of aldehydes to give carboxylic acids and alcohols. It is a 'disproportionation reaction' because the same compound undergoes both reduction and oxidation. In the following example of the reaction benzenecarbaldehyde is oxidized to benzenecarboxylic acid and reduced to benzene alcohol:
$2\ C_6H_5 CHO + H_2O = C_6H_5 COOH + C_6H_5 CH_2OH.$

c. True – if the soda lime is dry.

d. True – if the soda lime is dry.

e. True.

157 Answers

a. True – but the amount is negligible; see **154e**.

b. False – carbonyl chloride (phosgene) is a contaminant if TCE (trichloroethylene) is used. The agent is no longer in use and in any case it was incompatible with the use of soda lime for this very reason.

c. True.

d. False.

e. False.

158   Answers

a. **True.**
b. **False.**
c. **True.**
d. **True.**
e. **False.**

Note: if the cylinder contents are entirely gaseous then the Universal Gas equation – $PV = nRT$ – can be applied to determine their contents.

159   Answers

a. **True** – all oxygen cylinders, when full, have a pressure of 137 bar, no matter the cylinder size.
b. **True.**
c. **True.**
d. **True.**
e. **False** – about 50 bar.

160   Answers

a. **True.**
b. **True.**
c. **False.**
d. **True** – entonox cylinders are found with pin index outlets throughout the cylinder size range.
e. **False.**

161   Answers

a. **True** – the bevel is set obliquely to the shaft to make the needle tip blunt and thereby reduce the incidence of dural puncture.
b. **False** – the Murphy eye is a feature of tracheal tubes and urinary catheters (and some epidural needles: Braun Pencan) but not of the Tuohy needle.
c. **True** – the introducer device set in the hub of the needle facilitates threading the catheter.
d. **True** – a thin-walled needle with a straight blunt bevel without the curved Huber tip.
e. **True** – the wing at the junction of the shaft of the needle with its hub allows better control of needle advancement, the original one being the 'Weiss wing'.

162   Answers

a. **True.**
b. **True.**
c. **False.**
d. **True.**
e. **False** – triple cuff tube.

163 Answers

a. True.

b. False – of a lower refractive index.

c. False – coherence (i.e. precise geometric alignment) is not required if the purpose is merely to transmit light. It is necessary if a picture needs to be transmitted back to the endoscopist.

d. False – diameter of c. 20 micrometres.

e. True.

164 Answers

a. True.

b. False – at lease two atoms in the molecule but they need not be different.

c. True – because water vapour absorbs infrared radiations.

d. True – nitric oxide and nitrogen dioxide, both of which are paramagnetic.

e. True – needs a 0.6 V supply of electricity.

165 Answers

a. False.

b. True.

c. True.

d. False.

e. True.

Note: to be amenable to analysis by Raman scattering a gas must be at least di-atomic, though the atoms need not be of different elements.

166 Answers

a. False – because the gas molecules undergo ionization.

b. True.

c. True.

d. False – ultraviolet analysis is used for estimation of halothane, which is decomposed by it to form irritant byproducts.

e. True.

167 Answers

a. True – unless the instrument has been designed to accommodate water vapour estimation as well.

b. True.

c. True – because water vapour absorbs infrared light.

d. False.

e. False.

168   Answers

a. **False.**
b. **True.**
c. **False.**
d. **True.**
e. **False.**

Note: to be amenable to piezo-electric analysis, gases must be lipophilic.

169   Answers

a. **True** – the Beer–Lambert Law shows the relationship between the absorption of infrared energy and the concentration of the gas under test in accordance with the equation: $A = \log \frac{I_o}{I_e} = edC$, where A = absorption, I_o = incident intensity, I_e = exit intensity, e = molar extinction coefficient, d = length of path of travel, and C = sample concentration

b. **True.**
c. **False.**
d. **True** – because the absorption peak for CO_2 (4.26 μm) is very close to that for N_2O (4.5 μm). Analysers make provision for this phenomenon by including a correction factor.
e. **True** – because glass absorbs infrared radiations. Therefore the chamber windows are made of sapphire.

170   Answers

a. **True** – mass spectrometry can be used for all anaesthetic gases.
b. **False** – in volumes per cent units.
c. **False** – they cannot be returned because they have been ionized in the analytical process.
d. **False** – in direct proportion to their charge:mass ratio or in inverse proportion to their mass:charge ratio.
e. **True** – the flow must be very fine, i.e. molecular rather than viscous.

171   Answers

a. **False** – the agent must have at least two different elements in its molecule and therefore must at least be di-atomic.
b. **False** – for asymmetric polyatomic molecules.
c. **True.**
d. **False** – the sampled gases can be returned to patient breathing attachment because they have not undergone ionization.
e. **False.**

172 Answers

a. False – is a form of 'inelastic' scattering.
b. False – a partial transfer of energy from EMRs to matter.
c. True.
d. False.
e. False.

Note: *Scattering* of EMRs occurs when EMRs pass through a medium containing matter. In *elastic* scattering some of the radiations are reflected off the atoms and molecules without any change of energy. This type of scattering, also known as Rayleigh scattering, is associated with a change of phase but no change in frequency of the EMRs. In *inelastic* scattering interchange of energy occurs between the EMR photons and the particles, leading to a different wavelength and a different phase of the photons. Where the scattered radiations have a frequency higher than those of the incident radiations they are known as anti-Stokes radiations, when lower as Stokes radiations. Raman scattering is a type of inelastic scattering of light and ultraviolet radiation discovered by C V Raman in 1928. If a beam of monochromatic light is passed through a transparent substance some of the radiations will be scattered. Some of the scattered radiations will have frequencies above and some below those of the incident radiations. This production of radiations with altered frequencies is known as Raman scattering.

173 Answers

a. False.
b. False.
c. True.
d. True.
e. False.

174 Answers

a. True.
b. True.
c. True.
d. True.
e. True.

Note: all gases can be analysed by mass spectrometry.

175 Answers

a. True.
b. True.
c. True.
d. False.
e. False.

176 Answers

a. False – the haemoglobin concentration also needs to be known.
b. True – by reference to the HbO_2 dissociation curve.
c. False.
d. False – usually registers a high reading in the 90s.
e. False – shows a reading of c. 85%, irrespective of the actual amount of oxygen present combined with haemoglobin.

177 Answers

a. False – based on the presence of *unpaired* electrons in the outer orbit.
b. True.
c. True – the analyser readings depend on gas pressure within its cell which in turn is dependent on atmospheric pressure.
d. True – 'magnetic wind' is the alteration of the nonuniform magnetic field resulting from movement of the paramagnetic molecules into it.
e. True – nitric oxide and nitrogen dioxide.

178 Answers

a. False.
b. True – some paramagnetic analysers under-read oxygen by c. 1.5% in the presence of nitrous oxide.
c. True.
d. True.
e. False.

179 Answers

a. True – causes under-reading of CO_2 because of 'collision broadening'.
b. True – due to direct reduction of N_2O at the cathode when contaminated by Ag^+ ions from the reference electrode.
c. True – see **178b**.
d. False.
e. False.

180 Answers

a. True – by 'collision broadening', an intermolecular effect. Nitrous oxide increases the CO_2 signal.
b. True – by 'collision broadening', an intermolecular effect. Oxygen reduces the CO_2 signal.
c. False.
d. True – because glass absorbs infrared radiations.
e. False – sapphire is used instead of glass for the walls of the analyser chamber.

181 Answers

a. True – CO_2 is under-read if it is in a helium/oxygen mixture.
b. True.
c. True.
d. True.
e. True.

182 Answers

a. False – it does not generate its own electrical energy and therefore requires an extraneous energy source.
b. False – the measurement is in partial pressure units.
c. True.
d. True – affected by halothane.
e. True – $O_2 + 4e + 2H_2O = 4\ OH^-$.

183 Answers

a. False – neither has a platinum anode. Clark cell: platinum cathode and Ag/AgCl anode; fuel cell: lead anode and gold cathode.
b. False – neither has a lead cathode; see **a** above.
c. True – Clark cell: potassium chloride ; fuel cell: potassium hydroxide.
d. False – the Clark cell needs an external source of electricity; the fuel cell provides its own energy.
e. True – $O_2 + 4\ e + 2H_2O = 4OH^-$.

184 Answers

a. True.
b. False.
c. False.
d. False.
e. False.

185 Answers

a. True.
b. True – low drift voltages.
c. False – fragile electrodes.
d. False – because they contain silver the electrodes are prone to photosensitivity, which in turn can affect the 'half-cell' voltage.
e. True.

186 Answers

a. True.
b. False.
c. True.
d. False.
e. False.

187 Answers

a. False – SELV means 'safety extra low voltage' and is a phase supply whose voltage has been stepped down by means of a transformer.

b. True – RMS: 'root mean square'.

c. False – a 'line supply', rather than a phase supply, is more likely to be used in a radiology department for X-ray investigations because it combines two 'phase supplies'.

d. False – it is the common supply to households.

e. False – a lift needs a more powerful supply and therefore usually has a 'line supply'.

Note: mains electricity, when produced at the generating station, is a three-phase supply, i.e. three lots of electricity are produced from the same electromagnetic effect by using a single magnet but with three coils interposed between the poles of the magnet, the three coils being at 120 degrees to each other. Each coil produces one lot of electricity, the 'phase' supply. All three 'phases' are transmitted down the power cables for eventual supply to the consumer. In the case of domestic consumers, only one phase supply is required. In the case of heavier consumers, such as X-ray departments of hospitals, it is necessary to connect up two phase supplies to give a 'line' supply. In the case of industrial plants, it may be necessary to combine all three phase supplies together to provide the line supply.

188 Answers

a. False – other things being equal, a higher current threshold is required of a DC supply for inducing VF.

b. True.

c. False – there is no guarantee against electrocution other than by not using electricity. Even that may not save you, for you can be struck by lightning!

d. True.

e. False.

189 Answers

a. False – it is transmitted at high voltage (125 000–400 000 V) but at the standard frequency of 50 Hz.

b. True – about 3–3.5 MHz.

c. True – about 2–4 MHz so as to enable the production of an ultrasound wave of the same frequency.

d. False.

e. True – the use of frequencies near 30 MHz for heating is known as 'short wave diathermy'.

Answers

    a. False – note that the electricity, which can be battery provided, is required for setting the various ventilation parameters and operating the alarms. The energy for lung inflation is provided by pressurized gas, usually pipeline oxygen at 4 bar pressure.

    b. True – to maintain the desflurane vapour in the vaporizing chamber at a temperature of about 39 °C; a battery will not be able to supply sufficient heat energy for this purpose for any length of time. But there is a nonrechargeable battery incorporated in the vaporizer which provides power for the alarms and a liquid crystal level indicator during mains power failure.

    c. True.

    d. True – see **b** above.

    e. True – because it has to be a high frequency (3–3.5 MHz) alternating current.

191 **Answers**

    a. True – SELV: 'safety extra low voltage'. SELV may be DC or AC, but for cautery of warts the conventional mode is DC. This may be battery supplied or mains electricity suitably stepped down in voltage by a transformer and then rendered DC by means of a rectifier (diode).

    b. True.

    c. True.

    d. True – the magnetic field is maintained by passing electricity in a circuit rendered superconducting by being cooled to 4 K and then switching the current source off. At the extreme low temperature of 4 K there is no resistance to the flow of the (now) DC electricity and therefore no need for a potential difference.

    e. False – this needs AC electricity at the same frequency as the intended ultrasound wave.

192 **Answers**

    a. False – the galvanic cell generates its own potential difference.

    b. True.

    c. False – ISO regulations expressly state that the oxygen cut-off warning device shall be 'activated by oxygen and oxygen alone'.

    d. False.

    e. False.

193 **Answers**

    a. True.

    b. True.

    c. True.

    d. True.

    e. False – it is the work done when 1 m^3 of gas is moved against a pressure of 1 Pa.

194 Answers

a. False – about 1 ms.
b. True – about 10 microseconds.
c. False – 10–250 ms depending on the part of body being X-rayed.
d. False – 3–5 ms.
e. True – about 200–300 microseconds.

195 Answers

a. False – about 9 V.
b. True – c. 5000 V.
c. True – c. 3000–5000 V.
d. False – it is the usual 240 RMS voltage. It is the frequency that is higher, in the range of 2–4 MHz.
e. False.

196 Answers

a. True – 0.5–2.0 mV; typical amplitude 1 mV.
b. False – 5–200 μV; typical amplitude 50 μV.
c. True – 0.1–5 mV; typical amplitude 1 mV.
d. False – 0.5 mV.
e. False – 0.6 V.

197 Answers

a. True.
b. False – capacitance is measured in farads.
c. False – inductance is measured in henrys.
d. True.
e. True.

198 Answers

a. True – a current of about 50–80 mA.
b. True – threshold current for VF: 80–100 mA.
c. False – it is electrical energy; 200–360 J.
d. False – it is a voltage change that occurs with temperature change.
e. False – it is the 'current density', i.e. watts per unit surface area.

199 Answers

a. True.

b. True.

c. True.

d. False – if resistance is the only opposition to current flow in an AC circuit, then the voltage and current are in phase and therefore the resistance has a direct linear relationship with voltage. However, if there is a capacitor and/or inductor in the circuit, then the opposition to current flow is impedance. Since in such a circuit voltage and current are not in phase, the impedance will not bear a direct linear relationship to voltage.

e. True – if the only opposition to current flow is that of a resistor.

Note: *Impedance* in relation to electricity is a generic term for opposition to current flow in an AC circuit which has a resistor as well as a capacitor and/or inductor. The opposition to current flow in a resistor is *resistance*, and that in a capacitor or inductor is *reactance*. Therefore: impedance = resistance + reactance.

200 Answers

a. True – the other is resistance.

b. True.

c. True.

d. False – increases if there is an inductor in the circuit but decreases with increasing frequency if there is a capacitor in the circuit.

e. False – Z is the symbol for impedance, which is the sum of resistance and reactance.

201 Answers

a. False.

b. False – because no electricity will flow in a DC circuit which contains a capacitor. Therefore there can be no opposition to current 'flow' in it.

c. True.

d. True.

e. True.

202 Answers

a. False – Boyle temperature: the temperature at which a gas most closely resembles an ideal gas in its behaviour.

b. True – temperature at which a substance changes its magnetic properties.

c. True – Curie temperature (named after Pierre Curie): the temperature above which a ferromagnetic substance loses the property of ferromagnetism.

d. True – Neel temperature: the temperature above which an antiferromagnetic material becomes paramagnetic.

e. False – critical temperature: temperature above which a gas cannot be liquefied by pressure alone.

203 Answers

a. **True.**
b. **True.**
c. **False** – positive magnetic susceptibility.
d. **False** – magnetic domains are a feature of ferromagnetic materials.
e. **True.**

204 Answers

a. **True.**
b. **True.**
c. **False** – slightly less than one.
d. **False** – coercivity is a property of ferromagnetic materials.
e. **True** – hence a relative permeability of less than 1.

205 Answers

a. **True** – see **202c**.
b. **True.**
c. **True.**
d. **True** – remanence (or retentivity): the magnetic flux density remaining in a ferromagnetic substance when the saturating field is reduced to zero.
e. **True.**

206 Answers

a. **True.**
b. **False** – the purpose of a diathermy plate is *not* to provide a pathway for the diathermy current from the patient to earth; it is there to minimize the heating effect of the return pathway current at its interface with the patient's body and thereby reduce the current density to a level below the threshold that will cause a diathermy skin burn.
c. **False** – see **b** above.
d. **True.**
e. **True.**

207 Answers

a. **False** – 'isolated diathermy' and 'return electrode monitoring' are two separate and unrelated phenomena in relation to electrosurgery. An 'isolated' diathermy means that the system is isolated from earth and therefore no diathermy current can pass through the patient to earth. This arrangement minimizes the risk of electrocution from a 'leakage current'. The purpose of 'return electrode monitoring' is to ensure that there is sufficient apposition of the diathermy plate to the patient's skin at all times and thereby prevent the occurrence of a diathermy skin burn.
b. **True** – see **a** above.
c. **False** – 'cutting' diathermy normally requires the 'monopolar' mode and therefore a return electrical pathway and thus a diathermy plate. However, it need not to be an REM diathermy plate.
d. **True** – if bipolar diathermy is in use no diathermy plate, REM or 'ordinary', is necessary.
e. **False** – the mode of operation of the diathermy switch has no bearing on the type of diathermy plate required.

208 Answers

a. **True** – 'crest factor': ratio of peak voltage to the RMS voltage of the periodic waveform of AC electricity. In the case of 'cutting' diathermy the periodic waveform is a pure sine wave and the ratio is 1.4:1.0; in 'coagulation' diathermy, an on–off sine wave, the ratio is 3.0:1.0. The RMS voltage is the effective 'average' voltage over a period of time.

b. **True** – 'duty cycle': the ratio, expressed as a percentage, of the time for which a unit is activated to the total duration of the on–off cycle. In the case of 'cutting' diathermy the duty cycle is 100%, in 'coagulation' diathermy it is 5–10%. When a surgeon uses the 'blend' modality the duty cycle is about 50%.

c. **False** – cavitation is a phenomenon associated with ultrasound imaging.

d. **True** – channelling: the return of the diathermy current to the machine along an attenuated tissue pathway (such as a dissected and mobilized spermatic cord in a child during orchidopexy). This can lead to thermal damage to the cord because of the increased current density.

e. **False** – free induction decay is a phenomenon associated with MRI.

209 Answers

a. **True.**

b. **False.**

c. **True** – the radiofrequency signal must be of the same frequency as the resonant frequency of the precessing protons.

d. **True** – the piezo-electric crystal must be made of a material such that its resonant frequency matches that of the frequency of the ultrasound wave.

e. **False.**

210 Answers

a. **True.**

b. **True.**

c. **True.**

d. **False** – needs at least a battery supply.

e. **True** – can be operated off an oxygen cylinder employing the Bernoulli phenomenon and Venturi effect.

211 Answers

a. **True** – rectification: conversion of AC electricity to DC electricity by the use of a rectifier (diode).

b. **True** – an inductor in the defibrillator circuit helps 'level out' the current energy over the period of discharge into the patient. This enables a more successful cardioconversion with less thermal damage to the heart muscle.

c. **False** – remanence: a property of ferromagnetism.

d. **True** – the ability of a capacitor to store charge.

e. **False** – a phenomenon associated with the production of laser light energy.

212 Answers

a. **True.**
b. **True.**
c. **False.**
d. **False.**
e. **False.**

213 Answers

a. **True.**
b. **False** – it is a square within a square.
c. **True** – Class III equipment is SELV equipment: 'safety extra low voltage'.
d. **False** – lower maximum leakage current.
e. **False** – it reduces the risk of electrocution. There is no guarantee against electrocution other than doing away with the use of electricity.

214 Answers

a. **True.**
b. **False** – the symbol is a square within a square.
c. **True.**
d. **False** – it is AP or APG depending on whether it provides protection against ether and air mixtures or ether and oxygen mixtures; see **215c**.
e. **False** – the symbol is the letter F within a square.

215 Answers

a. **False** – Class I equipment is 'triple-wired', live, neutral and earthed.
b. **True** – Class II equipment is 'double insulated'.
c. **False** – ether and oxygen. It is AP equipment that provides protection against the most flammable mixture of ether and air.
d. **True** – SELV: 'safety extra low voltage'.
e. **False** – it is equipment that will not be damaged by the defibrillation current energy if it happens to be attached to a patient during defibrillation.

216 Answers

a. **True** – the purpose of a capacitor in a diathermy machine is to ensure that the machine will fail if the diathermy frequency falls below a certain level. The opposition to current flow in a capacitor diminishes with increasing frequency of the (alternating) current. Therefore if the frequency falls below a designated value the capacitor will oppose the flow of current, the machine will fail and the patient will be protected from the electrocuting effects of the lower frequency alternating current.
b. **True** – it stores the charge and has it ready for delivery through the heart muscle.
c. **True** – a capacitor, inductor or resistor can create the voltage change induced by pressure on the fluid coupled diaphragm.
d. **False.**
e. **False.**

217   Answers

   a. False – an oscillator is a device that converts DC electricity to AC
      electricity and therefore is not a necessary requirement for a mains
      (AC) powered defibrillator. It is however necessary for a battery
      powered defibrillator to convert the electricity from DC to AC so as
      to step up its voltage by means of a transformer (before it is re-
      converted to DC by means of a rectifier [diode]).
   b. True – a rectifier provides the opposite function to an oscillator; it
      converts AC electricity to DC; see **a** above.
   c. True – to step up the voltage from the mains (RMS) value of 230 to
      about 3000–5000 V.
   d. True – to help 'level out' the energy discharge during defibrillation.
   e. True – stores the energy just prior to its discharge through the
      patient.

218   Answers

   a. True – flow of an electric current in a circuit is in effect a flow of
      electrons in the opposite direction.
   b. True.
   c. False – it is the activity of protons that is imaged in MRI.
   d. True.
   e. False – it is the activity of photons resulting from the de-energizing
      electrons that makes the laser beam.

219   Answers

   a. False – Fink phenomenon (after Bernard Raymond Fink of Seattle):
      diffusion hypoxia seen at the end of a nitrous oxide anaesthetic when
      the patient is disconnected from the anaesthetic breathing attachment
      and then allowed to breathe room air.
   b. False – Cannizzaro reaction (after Stanislao Cannizzaro
      [1826–1910], the Italian chemist): a reaction of aldehydes to give
      carboxylic acids and alcohols, occurring as part of the chemical
      reactions between soda lime and halogenated inhalational anaesthetic
      agents.
   c. True – Larmor frequency (after Sir Joseph Larmor [1857–1942], the
      British physicist): the frequency of precession of the protons of
      hydrogen atoms when subjected to a magnetic field.
   d. False – Peltier effect (after Jean Peltier [1785–1845]): the change in
      temperature at the junction between two dissimilar metals or
      semiconductors when an electric current passes through the junction.
   e. False – Raman scattering (after Chandrasekara Raman [1880–1970]):
      a form of 'inelastic' scattering of light and ultraviolet radiation when a
      beam of monochromatic light is passed through a transparent
      medium.

220 Answers

a. **True** – 10% of the body mass is hydrogen. But because hydrogen is the lightest element, in molar terms it accounts for a much greater percentage – c. 63% – of the atoms in the body; 70% of the hydrogen in the body is in water, 20% in fat and the rest in protein.

b. **False** – although it is the lightest element it is its solitary proton that makes hydrogen unique as a signalling element for MRI; see **e** below.

c. **False** – hydrogen has two other isotopes, deuterium and tritium.

d. **False** – although forming hydrogen bonds, this property is not relevant in its role in MRI.

e. **True** – because it has a solitary proton in its nucleus.

221 Answers

a. **True.**
b. **False.**
c. **True.**
d. **False.**
e. **False.**

222 Answers

a. **True.**
b. **True.**
c. **True.**
d. **True.**
e. **True.**

223 Answers

a. **True** – production of heat in a conductor as a result of the passage of an electric current through it.

b. **True** – passage of an electric current through a conductor, the ends of which are maintained at different temperatures, results in heat being evolved in the conductor at a rate roughly proportional to the product of the current and the temperature gradient.

c. **False** – also known as the Joule–Thomson effect, it is the cooling resulting from adiabatic expansion of a gas.

d. **True** – generation of an EMF in a circuit containing two different metals (or semiconductors) when the junctions between the two are maintained at different temperatures.

e. **True** – change in temperature occurring at a junction of two dissimilar metals or semiconductors when an electric current passes through the junction. It is the opposite of the Seebeck effect.

224 Answers

a. **True** – it is what gives an element its unique identity.

b. **True** – it is the number of protons in an atom of the element.

c. **True.**

d. **True** – a neutral atom has an equal number of protons and electrons.

e. **False** – the isotope status of an element is determined by the atomic mass number, which is the nucleon number, i.e. the sum total of protons and neutrons in the nucleus of an atom of the element.

225 Answers

a. False – it is the mass of the 'dalton', which is the same as 1 atomic mass unit and is 1/12th of the mass of an atom of the isotope carbon-12 and is equal to 1.66033×10^{-27} kg. = *Avodagro number?*

b. True.

c. False – the number of electrons in a neutral atom is equal to the number of protons in that atom.

d. False – the symbol is A.

e. False – isotopes have the same atomic number but different atomic mass numbers.

226 Answers

a. True – London forces (also known as London dispersion forces and named after Fritz Wolfgang London [1900–1954] Polish–American physicist) are weak intermolecular forces that arise from the attractive force between transient dipoles in molecules without permanent multipole moments. London forces are one type of van der Waals forces.

b. False – a *hydrogen bond* is a type of attractive molecular force that exists between two partial electric charges of opposite polarity. It can exist between two parts of the same molecule, or between two adjacent molecules. While, as its name implies, a hydrogen atom forms one end of the bond, the other atom may be a strong electronegative element such as oxygen, nitrogen or fluorine.

c. False – hydrogen bonds are about 100 times stronger than dipole forces.

d. False – the presence of van der Waals forces detracts from the 'ideal gas' status of a gas.

e. False – the strongest are covalent bonds.

227 Answers

a. False – temporary dipole-dipole attractions.

b. False – weak forces.

c. True.

d. True – if van der Waals forces were not present, most substances would be permanently in the gaseous state.

e. True.

228 Answers

a. True.

b. False – are time-varying dipoles.

c. False – are weaker than hydrogen bonds.

d. True.

e. True – because they arise from uneven distribution of electrons within molecules, and larger molecules will have more electrons within them than will smaller molecules.

229 Answers

a. **False** – can form between any molecules as long as one of them has a hydrogen atom and the other has a strong electronegative element.
b. **False** – can also form between hydrogen and other electronegative elements.
c. **True** – many of the properties of water can be regarded as being due to the presence of hydrogen bonds.
d. **True.**
e. **True.**

230 Answers

a. **False** – they are strong dipole–dipole attractions, stronger than van der Waals attractions, and have about 10–20% of the energy of covalent bonds.
b. **True** – see **a** above.
c. **True.**
d. **True.**
e. **True** – the dielectric constant for water is about 80, the 'norm' being that for a vacuum, which is 1.

231 Answers

a. **True.**
b. **True.**
c. **True.**
d. **False** – it is an ionic bond between the phosphate moiety of 2,3 di-phosphoglyceraldehyde (2,3-DPG) and the amino acids of β-globin chains that helps link 2,3-DPG to haemoglobin.
e. **True** – by causing denaturing of bacterial cell wall proteins.

232 Answers

a. **True** – have a 'molar energy' of 356 kJ mol^{-1} for a C–C bond.
b. **False** – electron sharing is the feature of covalent bonding. Electron donation is the characteristic of ionic bonds.
c. **True** – if the two elements forming the covalent bond have different electronegativities then the sharing of electrons between them is 'asymmetrical', leading to 'polarity' between them.
d. **True** – a particular attribute, at their receptor sites, of irreversible antagonists of catecholamines and acetylcholine.
e. **False** – it is hydrogen bonds that have a role in DNA replication.

233 Answers

a. True – aspirin acts by attaching its acetyl group, by means of a covalent bond, to a serine residue in cyclo-oxygenase. This blocks the hydrophobic channel through which arachidonic acid reaches the active site of the enzyme.

b. False – ionic bonding; protamine sulphate is a low molecular weight cationic protein with two active binding sites. One helps protamine exert a mild anticoagulant effect of its own; the other binds to acidic polyanionic heparin to form a stable salt lacking any anticoagulant activity.

c. True – by combining with ferrous iron at the sixth coordination site.

d. True – hepatic metabolism of halothane involves its oxidation to trifluoroacetic acid – CF_3COOH – which reacts covalently with many proteins in liver cells, and the mechanism of hepatotoxicity is thought to involve an immune reaction to certain fluoroacetylated liver enzymes.

e. False – edrophonium is a short-acting quaternary ammonium compound that binds solely to the anionic site of the enzyme, compared with other anticholinesterases which bind to the esteratic site too. The binding is by means of an ionic bond and is readily reversible so that the action of edrophonium is very brief.

234 Answers

a. True.

b. False – an 'ideal' fluid is one that has no viscosity. It is a 'Newtonian fluid' that behaves in accordance with the Hagen–Poiseuille equation.

c. True – Raoult's Law: the partial vapour pressure of a solvent is proportional to its mole fraction of the solution. If p is the vapour pressure of the solvent and X the mole fraction of the solvent (i.e. the number of moles of solvent divided by the total number of moles of the solution), then $p = p_o X$, where p_o is the vapour pressure of the pure solvent.

d. False – a Newtonian fluid has a viscosity that is independent of its shear rate and its behaviour is in accordance with the Hagen–Poiseuille equation.

e. True.

235 Answers

a. True.

b. False – this is the Boyle temperature.

c. True.

d. True.

e. True – also known as the Curie temperature, after Pierre Curie.

236 Answers

a. False – Boyle temperature: the temperature at which a gas most closely approximates to an ideal gas.

b. True – see **235e**.

c. True – Neel temperature: the temperature above which an antiferromagnetic substance becomes paramagnetic.

d. False – colour temperature: the temperature to which a black body radiator must be raised so as to produce the same spectral distribution as the body in question.

e. False – critical temperature: the temperature above which a gas cannot be liquefied by pressure alone.

237 Answers

a. True.

b. False.

c. True.

d. True.

e. False.

Note: a colligative property is one that is dependent on the number of particles of the agent in question and not on its mass, size, charge or electrical activity.

238 Answers

a. True – Robert Boyle discovered the law in 1662. Edme Mariotte (1620–1684), the French physicist and plant physiologist, discovered it independently in 1676.

b. True.

c. True.

d. False – *Illuminance* and *luminance* are different from intensity of illumination. *Illuminance* indicates the degree of illumination of a surface lighting level of (say) a desk top surface or a surgical operation site. It is expressed in lumens per square metre ($lm\ m^{-2}$) or lux (lx) where 1 lx is 1 $lm\ m^{-2}$. *Luminance* is the measure of the amount of light arriving at a surface or emitted from or passing through it and its units are candela per square metre ($cd\ m^{-2}$). *Intensity of illumination* is a base quantity under the SI d'Unites and is measured in candela.

e. False – *cis–trans* isomerism is a form of structural isomerism and is also known as geometric isomerism. It is *keto-enol* tautomerism that is also known as dynamic isomerism.

239 Answers

a. True.
b. False – Bernoulli phenomenon: the law of conservation of mechanical energy (sum of kinetic and potential energy) as applied to the flow of fluids in tubes. Venturi effect: air entrainment at a constriction in a conduit during fluid flow, as a result of the fall of pressure resulting from a decrease in potential energy at that point.
c. True.
d. True.
e. True – because Sir William Thomson was later ennobled as Lord Kelvin.

240 Answers

a. True.
b. True.
c. True.
d. False.
e. False.

241 Answers

a. True.
b. False – D- and L-isomerism is one system of nomenclature for enantiomers (the other is the *R* and *S* nomenclature), and is so named by reference to the Fischer projection for the two enantiomers of glyceraldehyde. *d*- and *l*-isomers, on the other hand, are named in accordance with the direction of rotation of plane polarized light, *d* (dextro-rotatory) and *l* (laevorotatory).
c. True.
d. False – conformers are different conformations of the *same* molecule; configurational isomers are *different* molecules.
e. True.

242 Answers

a. False – a racemic mixture is a 50:50 mixture of two enantiomers. It exhibits no optical activity because the rotation of light in one direction by one enantiomer is cancelled by rotation in the opposite direction by the other.
b. False – it is also possible when a carbon–carbon single bond (C–C) is present in a ring structure.
c. False – they also differ in respect of optical activity, rotating plane-polarized light in opposite directions.
d. False.
e. True.

243 Answers

a. True.
b. False – two enantiomers rotate plane polarized light in opposite directions but their degrees of rotation are the same.
c. False.
d. False.
e. False.

244 Answers

a. **True.**
b. **False** – *cis–trans* isomers are one type of stereo-isomer, often called diastereomers, to distinguish them from a second type of stereo-isomer viz. enantiomers.
c. **False** – can occur in single-bond carbon atoms if they are part of a ring structure, e.g. a benzene ring.
d. **True** – configuration: spatial orientation in which the substituents extend out from the carbon atoms into the planes on opposite sides of the carbon atoms.
e. **False** – *keto-enol* isomerism is a feature associated with thiopentone activity.

245 Answers

a. **True.**
b. **True.**
c. **True.**
d. **True.**
e. **True.**

Note: because they are mirror images, enantiomers differ from one another only with respect to mirror-image properties viz. rotation of plane-polarized light. Diastereomers, on the other hand, are not mirror images of one another; they may differ in all properties, chiral or achiral, including the number of degrees by which they rotate plane-polarized light. In short, they behave as two different chemical substances.

246 Answers

a. **False.**
b. **False.**
c. **False.**
d. **True.**
e. **False** – although enantiomeric isomers differ in their *direction* of rotation of plane-polarized light, they show the same specific rotation of light.

247 Answers

a. **False** – consists of a 50:50 mixture of two stereo-isomers.
b. **True.**
c. **False.**
d. **True.**
e. **False.**

248 Answers

a. **False** – it is a type of structural isomerism.
b. **False** – *cis–trans* isomerism is the same as geometric isomerism.
c. **True** – different spatial orientation of the substituents.
d. **False** – they also differ in respect of optical activity, rotating plane-polarized light in opposite directions.
e. **False** – they are structural isomers.

249 Answers

a. **False** – may be a *diastereomer*.
b. **True.**
c. **False.**
d. **True.**
e. **False.**

250 Answers

a. **True** – *cis–trans* isomerism (also known as geometric isomerism) is one form of stereo-isomerism, the other being optical isomerism.
b. **False** – is a form of structural isomerism, like *keto–enol* isomerism. It is not a form of stereo-isomerism.
c. **True** – rotamers are compounds that are each convertible to the other by rotation about a carbon–carbon bond.
d. **False** – constitutional isomerism is the same as structural isomerism.
e. **True** – configurational isomers are stereo-isomers that can be interconverted only by breaking and re-making bonds; e.g. in the case of *cis–trans* isomers in alkenes or cycloalkanes.

251 Answers

a. **False** – almost all.
b. **True** – usually do.
c. **True** – typically contain 14–24 carbon atoms, most commonly between 16 and 18.
d. **True.**
e. **True.**

252 Answers

a. **False** – the opposite of resistance is conductance; elastance is the opposite of compliance.
b. **True** – see **a** above; whether it is electricity or gas flows, the same applies.
c. **False** – Joule–Kelvin effect is the same as Joule–Thomson effect, viz. adiabatic decompression. Sir William Thomson was ennobled as Lord Kelvin.
d. **False** – Joule effect: liberation of heat from a conductor when a current flows in it (note: the heat is produced irrespective of the direction of current flow). Peltier effect: occurs when current is passed through a single junction between two dissimilar conductors; heat is liberated or absorbed depending on the direction of the current.
e. **True** – Bohr effect: the enhanced oxygen release by haemoglobin in the presence of a low pH. It normally occurs in systemic capillaries. Haldane effect: the opposite of the Bohr effect, occurs in the pulmonary capillaries; as the oxygen-binding by haemoglobin increases, the latter's CO_2-carrying capacity falls.

253 Answers

a. **False** – *keto–enol* tautomerism is the same as dynamic isomerism; *cis–trans* isomerism is the same as geometric isomerism.

b. **False** – ohm: unit of electrical resistance; siemens: unit of electrical conductance, also known as the mho.

c. **True** – atomic mass unit: a unit of mass equal to 1/12th of the mass of the carbon-12 atom and equal to 1.66033×10^{-27} kg.

d. **True** – also known as the Kelvin scale.

e. **True** – named after Lambert Adolphe Quetelet (1796–1874), the Belgian astronomer and statistician.

254 Answers

a. **False** – stress relaxation: the ability of smooth muscle (especially in the case of a hollow viscus) to return nearly to its original force of contraction within seconds or minutes after it has been elongated or shortened. Latch phenomenon: low energy consumption–high tension state: ability of smooth muscle to maintain a high force (tone) for long periods but at a low rate of energy consumption (ATP hydrolysis). The two phenomena although different are nevertheless closely related.

b. **True** – the ability of a structure to be both hydrophobic and hydrophilic. The cell membrane is such a structure.

c. **False** – amphotericity: the property of a substance to react chemically either as an acid or an alkali. Water is amphoteric because it dissociates into H^+ (acid) and OH^- (alkali). Amino acids too are amphoteric because they can act both as acids ($-COO^-$) and as bases (NH_4^+). Amphibolicity: the ability of a series of chemical reactions to proceed in either direction. The Krebs tricarboxylic acid cycle is the paradigm example.

d. **False** – luminance: luminous intensity per unit area arriving at or leaving a surface or passing through it in a given direction. It is expressed in lumens per square metre per steradian. Illuminance: luminous power density incident on a surface. It is expressed in lumens per square metre or lux. Luminance = illuminance $\times$ reflectance.

e. **False** – *R*-, *S*-isomerism is determined by reference to the configuration of the stereogenic centre of the isomer. The four groups attached to the stereogenic centre are placed in an order of priority and the centre is then observed from the side opposite the lowest priority. If the three remaining groups form a clockwise array, the configuration is designated *R* (Latin: *rectus*: right), if they form a counterclockwise array, it is designated *S* (Latin: *sinister*: left). *d*-, *l*-isomerism (not to be confused with the D- and L- forms of substances) refers to the observed rotation of polarized light by the substance.

255 Answers

a. **True** – because it is a colligative property.

b. **False.**

c. **False.**

d. **True** – because this will lead to an increase in the number of particles.

e. **False.**

256 Answers

a. True – it is the joule.
b. True – newtons per square metre, i.e. pascals.
c. False – compliance: litres per centimetre water pressure; conductance: centimetres water pressure per unit flow rate, i.e. litres per second.
d. False – luminance: lumens per square metre per steradian or candela per steradian; illuminance: lumens per square metre, which is the same as lux.
e. False – dynamic viscosity: newton seconds per square metre or pascal seconds; former non-SI unit: poise. Kinematic viscosity is dynamic viscosity divided by density and therefore has the SI units metres^2 per second. The former (cgs) unit is the stokes, where 1 stokes is equal to 1 cm^2 s^{-1}.

257 Answers

a. True.
b. False.
c. False.
d. True.
e. True.

258 Answers

a. True.
b. True.
c. False – 'temperature compensation' in relation to a TEC vaporizer does not mean that the temperature of the vaporizing chamber remains unchanged. It means that if there is a fall in temperature, and therefore a reduction in the amount of agent vaporized, the vaporizer will compensate for the change by restoring the amount vaporized to its original level so as to maintain the concentration of agent in the exit carrier gases the same.
d. False – the boiling point of a liquid is the temperature at which its saturation vapour pressure equals ambient pressure. Therefore, for instance, at the top of Mount Everest, where the ambient pressure is about 35 kPa, the boiling point of water will be about 80°C because the SVP of water at 80°C is about 35 kPa.
e. True.

259 Answers

a. True.
b. True.
c. True – and thus reduce the current density (watts per centimetre^2) below the threshold likely to cause a diathermy burn under the plate.
d. False – to reduce the degree of acoustic mismatch at the probe–skin interface.
e. True.

260 Answers

a. False – opposition to current flow through an inductor (known as 'reactance') has a direct linear relationship with the frequency of the alternating current; opposition to current flow in a capacitor is inversely related to frequency.
b. False – its propagation is rendered more difficult.
c. False – it is higher.
d. True.
e. False – the risk is higher because the energy of EMRs is directly proportional to their frequency. But the risk of *electrical* injury, i.e. electrocution, is lower.

261 Answers

a. False – graded according to their diameter in millimetres.
b. False – graded as small, medium and large.
c. False – according to SWG (steel wire gauge).
d. True.
e. False – according to SWG.

Note: FCG grading is according to the external circumference in millimetres.

262 Answers

a. False – orotracheal tubes are graded according to their diameter in millimetres.
b. False – graded according to their diameter in millimetres.
c. True – numbers 35, 37, 39 and 41.
d. False – the grading is 'arbitrary' numbering.
e. False – the grading is 'arbitrary' numbering.

263 Answers

a. False – according to the diameter in millimetres.
b. True.
c. True.
d. False – quadruple lumen central venous catheters are now graded according to FCG.
e. True.

Note: SWG (steel wire gauge) is a 'dimensionless entity'; it refers to the number of steel wires of the same diameter as the device in question that can be accommodated inside a standard hollow cylinder. Therefore the higher the SWG number, the smaller the size of the device.

264 Answers

a. **True.**
b. **False.**
c. **True.**
d. **False.**
e. **False.**

Note: Murphy eye: introduced into orotracheal tubes by Frank J Murphy of the Department of Anesthesiology, Harper Hospital, Detroit, Michigan in 1941.

265 Answers

a. **True** – in Boyle's Law the constant is temperature, i.e. the change is isothermal and has to be so to render the law valid.
b. **False** – in Charles' Law one of the variables is temperature (the other is volume).
c. **False** – Gay-Lussac's Law depicts a linear relationship between pressure and thermodynamic temperature of a fixed mass of gas at constant volume.
d. **False** – it *is* the change in pressure that is being measured.
e. **True.**

266 Answers

a. **False** – potential energy increases.
b. **True** – potential energy of the coiled spring is converted into kinetic energy.
c. **True** – because potential energy needs to be converted to kinetic energy in accordance with the Bernoulli equation.
d. **True** – as an object falls from a height its velocity must increase owing to the gravitational pull of the earth. Therefore its kinetic energy must increase and, therefore, in accordance with the law of conservation of mechanical energy, its potential energy must decrease.
e. **True** – because energy needs to be expended to overcome the van der Waals attractions between the gas molecules, and this is the reason for the drop in temperature.

267 Answers

a. **True.**
b. **False** – it is 100 000 (10^5) Pa.
c. **False** – it is 10 000 000 Å.
d. **True.**
e. **False** – it is about 140 000 Hz.

268 Answers

a. **True.**
b. **True** – 1 centilitre = 10 ml.
c. **True.**
d. **False** – it is 10 000 dynes cm^{-2}.
e. **False** – it is 100 pm in 1 Å.

269 Answers

a. True – I atmosphere = 10 mH$_2$0 pressure = 1000 cmH$_2$O pressure.
b. False – 10 000 gauss = 1 T.
c. True – because the solution has 1 mmol ml^{-1}.
d. False – it is 760 torr in 1 bar (1 torr = 1 mmHg).
e. True.

270 Answers

a. True.
b. True – 1 Gy = 100 rads.
c. True – 1 Sv = 100 rems.
d. False – 10 Å = 1 nm.
e. False – 10 cmH$_2$O pressure = 1 kPa.

271 Answers

a. True.
b. True.
c. False – 1 mmHg = 1.36 cmH$_2$O pressure.
d. False – 100 pm = 1 Å.
e. True.

272 Answers

a. True – variable, but an average figure of 10 kilo-ohms is about right.
b. True – produced at a generating station at c. 25 000 V and transmitted at voltages between 125 000 and 400 000 V.
c. False – it is c. 2.5 GHz.
d. True – c. 140 000 Hz.
e. True – about 250 kilo-ohms.

273 Answers

a. True.
b. True.
c. False.
d. True.
e. True.

274 Answers

a. True.
b. True – at its resonant frequency the reactance of a capacitor and that of an inductor cancel each other out. So, the only opposition to flow of electric current would be the resistance of a resistor in the circuit, and therefore the current would be maximal.
c. True – the radiofrequency wave during MRI should be the same as that of the hydrogen protons, i.e. at its resonant frequency.
d. True – this will enable the ultrasound waves to be at 'full strength' and thereby enhance their effects.
e. False.

275 Answers

a. True.
b. True – reduces the risk of explosion.
c. True.
d. False.
e. False.

276 Answers

a. True – because the relationship is inverse: $i \propto \dfrac{1}{R}$; $(V = iR)$. Wherever there is an : $A \propto \dfrac{1}{B}$ relationship, its graphical representation takes the form of a rectangular hyperbola, e.g. pressure and volume according to Boyle's Law.
b. False – if the increase in specific gravity is due to an increase in the protein content, then specific gravity will increase at a disproportionately greater rate than osmolarity.
c. False – blood is a thixotropic fluid, i.e. its viscosity varies inversely with the velocity of blood flow.
d. False – not in the case of laser light, because it is 'collimated'.
e. True – many of the properties of water (high boiling point, high dielectric constant, higher density than ice, etc.) are due to the fact that it has a high dipole moment and this in turn is due to the presence of hydrogen bonds in the water molecule.

277 Answers

a. False – heating a liquid for any length of time needs a large amount of electrical energy, which can be provided effectively only by means of a mains AC supply or suitable AC alternative (generator).
b. True – the gas delivery is effected by a driving gas (usually oxygen) at a pressure of 4 bar. Electricity is required to operate the various ventilatory parameter controls and this can be done with a battery supply.
c. True – this is done manually.
d. True – by use of pressurized gases (e.g. O_2 at 4 bar pressure) and application of the Bernoulli phenomenon and Venturi effect.
e. True – by use of a low voltage 6–12 V DC battery electric current.

278 Answers

a. False – 'plenum' and 'TEC' are two different attributes of a vaporizer and serve two different functions. In a 'plenum' vaporizer, as opposed to a draw-over vaporizer, the carrier gases always flow under positive pressure and therefore the pressure in the vaporizer never falls below ambient pressure (cf. a draw-over vaporizer in which the pressure never rises above ambient pressure). A 'TEC' vaporizer is a 'temperature compensated' vaporizer, the compensation effect being produced by the bimetallic strip sited in the bypass chamber.
b. True.
c. False – although the Manley MP 3 ventilator, which is a constant pressure generator ventilator, is in fact a minute volume divider.
d. True – so as to convert AC (mains) electricity into DC electricity.
e. False – it may be made into a low-flow ('re-breathing') attachment by incorporating a soda lime canister in the circuitry.

279   Answers

a. True – because the DC voltage of the battery (may be about 12 V) must be stepped up to several kilovolts. This can only be done by means of a transformer, and step-up or step-down of electrical voltage can only be done with AC electricity. Therefore the DC electricity must first be converted to AC by means of an oscillator, then stepped-up and then re-converted to DC by means of a rectifier (diode).

b. False – there is no need for a pressure regulator because the pipeline supply is already at a pressure of about 4 bar.

c. False – the heating of fluids cannot be done satisfactorily with low voltage current; it needs a (240 V) mains AC electricity supply. So there is no place for a step-down transformer.

d. False – although TEC Mark 4 vaporizers normally have a large heatsink it is not an essential pre-requisite for the vaporizer's performance. 'Temperature compensation' is provided by the bimetallic strip in the bypass chamber.

e. True – preferably in DC form. (SELV: safety extra-low voltage).

280   Answers

a. False – kinetic energy is converted into potential energy.

b. False – kinetic energy is converted into potential energy.

c. True.

d. True.

e. False – conversion of mechanical energy (both kinetic and potential) into electrical energy.

281   Answers

a. True – channelling: the tendency of the diathermy electric current to seek a return pathway to the electrosurgical (diathermy) unit through attenuated tissue such as a dissected and mobilized spermatic cord. This results in a high 'current density' in the cord and thermal injury to the tissue. Therefore, the bipolar mode is the appropriate one.

b. False – the phenomenon is 'cavitation', the formation of microbubbles in tissues from the high peak pressures caused by the US waves. If they were to subsequently expand to the point of very sudden collapse they can cause a huge rise in tissue temperature and consequent tissue damage.

c. True – bypassing of the soda lime by the exhaled anaesthetic gases with consequent nonremoval of its CO_2.

d. True – the mechanism of production is the same as explained in **a**.

e. False – the phenomenon is 'precession'.

282   Answers

a. **True.**
b. **False.**
c. **False.**
d. **True** – the fibrelight fibres need to maintain the same geometric alignment to each other throughout the full length of the fibre-optic cable.
e. **True.**

Note: coherence is (i) the propagation of waves in the same phase with respect to amplitude and (ii) maintaining the same geometric alignment throughout the length of cable.

283   Answers

a. **True.**
b. **True.**
c. **True.**
d. **False** – 7 bar line pressure.
e. **False** – the 'opening' pressure is about 40 kPa.

284   Answers

a. **False.**
b. **True.**
c. **False.**
d. **False.**
e. **False.**

285   Answers

a. **True** – $f \propto \frac{1}{\lambda}$.
b. **False** – the reciprocal of resistance is conductance; that of compliance is elastance.
c. **True.**
d. **False** – dielectric constant and relative permittivity are one and the same.
e. **False** – permeability: ratio of the magnetic flux density in a substance to the external field strength; coercivity: the magnetizing force required to reduce the magnetic flux density in a ferromagnetic material to 0.

286   Answers

a. **False** –unlike α particles (positive charge) and β particles (negative charge), γ rays do not possess a charge.
b. **True** – because they have a higher frequency than X-rays, and the energy of EMRs is directly proportional to their frequencies.
c. **True** – because they are EMRs, and all EMRs travel at the speed of light.
d. **False** – have a weak ability to produce fluorescence, unlike α particles which are capable of strong fluorescence.
e. **True** – all (noncollimated) EMRs obey the inverse square law in this regard.

287 Answers

a. **True** – the reading is invariably in the upper 90s, irrespective of the actual haemoglobin oxygen saturation.
b. **True.**
c. **True.**
d. **False** – it would be lower.
e. **True** – because nitric oxide is a paramagnetic gas.

288 Answers

a. **True.**
b. **True.**
c. **True.**
d. **True.**
e. **True.**

289 Answers

a. **False** – heat energy can be transmitted by radiation, although not by conduction, convection or evaporation.
b. **True.**
c. **True.**
d. **False.**
e. **True.**

290 Answers

a. **True** – this is Wien's Law.
b. **True.**
c. **False** – it is a direct relationship.
d. **True.**
e. **True.**

291 Answers

a. **True** – $\omega \propto B_0$, where ω = angular frequency in radians, B_0 = static magnetic field in tesla. Therefore, $\omega = \gamma B_0$ (where γ is the gyromagnetic ratio).
b. **False** – inverse relationship; the lower the Michaelis constant the greater an enzyme's affinity for its substrate.
c. **True** – the higher the AC frequency the greater the reactance in an inductor in the circuit.
d. **False** – there is no constant relationship between the density of a liquid and its viscosity.
e. **False** – the lower the blood–gas partition coefficient, the faster the rate of anaesthetic induction.

292 Answers

a. **True.**
b. **False** – it is a sine wave.
c. **False** – traditionally it was a damped sine wave, but the modern form can be monophasic or biphasic, and each of these may be 'sawtoothed', 'rectilinear' or truncated'.
d. **False.**
e. **False.**

293 Answers

a. **False** – the pattern is a sine wave.
b. **True.**
c. **True.**
d. **False** – it is a sine wave.
e. **True.**

294 Answers

a. **True.**
b. **True.**
c. **True.**
d. **True** – nitric oxide and nitrogen dioxide are also paramagnetic, but NO is not used in significant quantities and NO_2 is not present at all in medical gas mixtures.
e. **True** – it has an absorption spectrum at about 200 nm.

295 Answers

a. **True** – aspirin is an example.
b. **True** – digoxin, chloramphenicol are examples.
c. **True** – heparin (negatively charged), and tubocurarine and suxamethonium (positively charged) are examples.
d. **False** – it depends on the respective electronegativities of the bonded atoms; if they are the same, the molecule will have absolute electro-equivalence; if different, the molecule will be polar, the degree of polarity depending on the respective electronegativities of the atoms of the molecule.
e. **False** – weak dipole–dipole attractions.

296 Answers

a. **True.**
b. **False** – this is the transition temperature.
c. **False** – this is its Boyle temperature.
d. **True.**
e. **False.**

Note: Curie temperature is named after Pierre Curie.

297 Answers

a. **True.**
b. **True.**
c. **True.**
d. **False.**
e. **False.**

298 Answers

a. True.
b. False – relates to precessing protons.
c. True.
d. False.
e. True.

Note: Larmor frequency: the frequency of precession of protons in a nucleus. In the case of MRI the nucleus is that of the hydrogen atom.

299 Answers

a. False.
b. False.
c. False.
d. True.
e. False.

300 Answers

a. False – cavitation: the formation, growth and then violent collapse of gas bubbles during, respectively, the rarefaction and compression stages of an ultrasound pressure wave cycle. Such alterations can lead to both physical damage to and chemical change in body tissues.
b. False – channelling (i) in diathermy: the return of the diathermy current to the machine along an attenuated tissue pathway (such as a dissected and mobilized spermatic cord in a child during orchidopexy). This can lead to thermal damage to the cord because of the increased current density; (2) in a breathing attachment: the bypassing of soda lime by expired gases in a low flow circle breathing attachment (leading to re-breathing of exhaled CO_2).
c. True – collimation: nondivergence of a light beam in its propagation. Therefore laser light does not obey the inverse square law with respect to distance of transmission.
d. True – population inversion: the presence of a higher percentage of particles of the lasing medium in the excited state than in the ground state.
e. False – precession is a phenomenon associated with MRI.

301 Answers

a. True – acoustic impedance: opposition of a medium to the flow of sound energy waves (cf. electrical impedance). The *specific acoustic impedance* of a medium is the product of the density of the medium and the velocity of sound in it.
b. False – superconductivity is a phenomenon relating to MRI scanning.
c. True – coherence is the presence of a constant phase relationship during propagation of waves so that peaks and troughs of waves are similarly spaced. This is what it is intended will happen to sound waves created by a piezo-electric crystal so that their amplitudes are additive and they thus retain – and accentuate – their sound energies.
d. False – graded index transmission is a phenomenon of fibre-optic transmission.
e. False – gyromagnetic ratio: ratio of angular frequency (ω) of spinning protons to the external magnetic field (B_o) in MRI scanning.

302   **Answers**

   a. False.
   b. True.
   c. True – this is why ships' foghorns are of low pitch, so that they can be heard better at greater distances.
   d. False – energy level is proportional to the square of its amplitude.
   e. True – can lead to 'cavitation', which is accompanied by heating of tissues.

303   **Answers**

   a. False – thermal jostling occurs in MRI. It is the 'competition' of the electron dipoles of hydrogen atoms for energy imparted to them by the applied magnetic field, causing those with less energy to align themselves in the direction of the field (parallel or 'spin up') and those with more energy to align in a direction opposite to the magnetic field (antiparallel or 'spin down').
   b. True – acoustic mismatch: a marked difference in the specific acoustic impedances of two media at their interface, leading to reflection of a major fraction of the ultrasound wave.
   c. False – coercivity: a feature of ferromagnetism. It refers to the magnetizing force required to reduce the magnetic flux density in a magnetic material to 0.
   d. True – the amount of the sound wave reflected back at the interface of two media as a fraction of that incident on the interface.
   e. False – spin–spin interaction is a phenomenon associated with MRI.

304   **Answers**

   a. True.
   b. True.
   c. False – remanence is a phenomenon of ferromagnetism.
   d. False – spin-lattice relaxation is a phenomenon of MRI.
   e. False – collimation (nondivergence of a light beam during its propagation) is a phenomenon associated with laser light.

Practice paper 1

1.1 The following are fundamental units under the SI units system:

   a. Metre.
   b. Ampere.
   c. Radian.
   d. Second.
   e. Gram.

1.2 The following are non-SI units:

   a. Siemens.
   b. Stokes.
   c. Gray.
   d. Electron-volt.
   e. Poise.

1.3 The steradian:

   a. Is a dimensionless entity.
   b. Is a fundamental unit under the SI units system.
   c. Is the unit of plane angle.
   d. Is a necessary component in the measurement of luminance.
   e. Is a necessary component in the definition of the unit of lumen.

1.4 The following 'quantities' are ratings, i.e. their units indicate the rate at which the particular physical phenomenon occurs:

   a. Electric current.
   b. Power.
   c. Illuminance.
   d. Resistance (in relation to flow of a fluid in a conduit).
   e. Capacitance.

1.5 The following statements are true:

   a. The ampere is the unit of quantity of electrical energy.
   b. The lumen is the unit of quantity of light energy.
   c. The watt is the unit of quantity of heat energy.
   d. The poise is the unit of kinematic viscosity.
   e. The tesla is the unit of magnetic flux.

1.6 The following are dimensionless entities:

   a. Extinction coefficient (in relation to light).
   b. Temperature coefficient of resistance (in relation to electricity).
   c. Damping coefficient.
   d. Diffusion coefficient.
   e. Permeability coefficient (of cell membrane).

1.7 The inverse square law correctly applies to the following:

a. Intensity of collimated light in relation to distance of propagation.
b. Intensity of X-rays and their distance from source.
c. Magnitude of van der Waals forces between two atoms and the distance separating them.
d. Laminar flow rate of a fluid and the cross-sectional area of the tube.
e. Total intensity of emitted radiations of a 'perfect black body' and its Kelvin temperature.

1.8 The following processes, when graphically depicted, take the form of an exponential decay:

a. Disintegration of a radionuclide.
b. Volume change of a fixed mass of gas in accordance with Charles' Law.
c. Pressure change of a fixed mass of gas in accordance with Gay-Lussac's Law.
d. Variation of light intensity in accordance with the Beer–Lambert Law.
e. Voltage of a discharging capacitor in a DC electrical circuit.

1.9 The following have the mathematical relationship $A \propto B^2$:

a. The molecular weight of a substance and its rate of passive diffusion down its concentration gradient.
b. The kinetic energy of a gas and the mean velocity of its molecules.
c. The electrical energy in a system and the current flowing in it.
d. The radiation energy emitted by a body and its Kelvin temperature.
e. Intensity of a beam of light and the amplitude of its wave.

1.10 In the case of time constant:

a. It is a phenomenon of zero-order activity systems.
b. It is shorter than the half-life of the particular system.
c. It is mathematically equal to resistance × compliance for the lungs.
d. Mathematically, it could be equal to the product of electrical resistance and capacitance.
e. It is mathematically equal to electrical inductance multiplied by electrical resistance.

1.11 In the case of an 'ideal gas':

a. It conforms to Boyle's Law.
b. It conforms to Charles' Law.
c. It conforms to Gay-Lussac's Law.
d. It conforms to Avogadro's Law.
e. The speed of sound in it is temperature related.

1.12 **An adiabatic change of state:**

a. Can be described as the Joule–Thomson effect.
b. Will render Boyle's Law invalid.
c. Usually occurs when the oxygen cylinder of an anaesthetic machine empties.
d. Occurs in the functioning of the cryoprobe.
e. Can be associated with a risk of fire.

1.13 **In the case of a Newtonian fluid:**

a. Its flow rate is independent of its shear stress.
b. The resistance to flow in a conduit is in accordance with the hydraulic form of Ohm's Law.
c. The relationship between flow rate and cross-sectional area of conduit is in accordance with the inverse square law.
d. Both viscosity and density are operational factors in determining flow rate.
e. Its flow rate has a direct linear relationship with pressure gradient.

1.14 **The Venturi effect (creation of a 'negative' pressure in a fluid flow system) prevails in the performance of the following devices:**

a. Co-axial Bain attachment during spontaneous ventilation.
b. Suction apparatus operated by means of pressurized oxygen.
c. Nebulizer used for humidification of inspired gases.
d. Pitot tube.
e. Sanders injector during 'jet ventilation' at bronchoscopy.

1.15 **The following devices determine temperature by measuring a dimensional change in matter:**

a. Mercury clinical thermometer.
b. Alcohol thermometer.
c. Bimetallic strip thermometer.
d. Bourdon gauge thermometer.
e. Infrared thermometer.

1.16 **The following temperature measuring devices show a linear change of the particular parameter over the conventional operational range with change in temperature:**

a. Platinum resistance thermometer.
b. Thermistor.
c. Mercury clinical thermometer.
d. Gas thermometer.
e. Thermocouple.

1.17 The following methods of gas analysis monitor the agents by determining partial pressure rather than their volumes per cent in the mixture:

a. Mass spectrometry.
b. Raman scattering.
c. Infrared analysis.
d. Ultraviolet analysis.
e. Piezo-electric method.

1.18 Gaseous oxygen can be measured by the following methods:

a. Mass spectrometry.
b. Infrared analysis.
c. Ultraviolet analysis.
d. Raman scattering.
e. Paramagnetic analysis.

1.19 In gas analysis by mass spectrometry:

a. The monitor must necessarily be programmed only for those gases it is intended to estimate.
b. Measurement is on a volumes per cent basis rather than in partial pressure units.
c. Analysis response time is fast enough for reliable end-tidal measurements of gases.
d. It is essential to ionize the gases prior to analysis.
e. The method cannot analyse mono-atomic gaseous agents.

1.20 Nitrous oxide can be assayed by the following methods of gas analysis:

a. Mass spectrometry.
b. Raman scattering.
c. Infrared gas analysis.
d. Paramagnetic analysis.
e. Piezo-electric method of gas analysis.

1.21 The presence of the following are recognized as adversely affecting the accuracy of conventional pulse oximetry:

a. Prominent venous pulsations at the sampling site.
b. Methylene blue in the blood.
c. Fluorescein dye in the circulation.
d. Henna, a finger and toe stain, at the sampling site.
e. Dried blood at the sampling site.

1.22 The operational electric current in the following situations is of the order of milliamperes rather than amperes:

a. Current that induces ventricular fibrillation.
b. Current used for synchronized DC cardioconversion.
c. PNS current for double burst stimulation.
d. Current used in the TENS (transcutaneous electrical nerve stimulation) machine.
e. Electrosurgical current used during a TUR of the prostate gland.

1.23 The following devices perform their function by detecting a change in electrical impedance:

a. Platinum resistance thermometer.
b. Interrogation current of an REM diathermy return electrode plate.
c. A fluid-coupled transducer device for invasive arterial blood pressure measurement.
d. Thermocouple used for temperature measurement.
e. A piezo-electric crystal when used for producing ultrasound.

1.24 The following statements are true with respect to electricity:

a. A potential difference is always necessary if current is to flow in an electrical circuit.
b. In a pure resistor AC circuit, voltage and current are in phase.
c. Reactance in a circuit is the aggregate of impedance, resistance and inductance.
d. The current is maximal in an AC circuit when it is at resonant frequency.
e. The risk of VF from a faulty appliance is greater if it is energized by direct current rather than alternating current.

1.25 The electrical stimulus pattern of each of the following devices is in the nature of a 'square-wave' pulse:

a. Discharge current of a conventional DC defibrillator.
b. Train-of-Four current of a peripheral nerve stimulator.
c. 'Cutting mode' current of an isolated diathermy (electrosurgical) unit.
d. Cardiac pacemaker current.
e. Stimulus of a TENS (transcutaneous electrical nerve stimulation) apparatus.

1.26 For reasons of safety and/or of accuracy of performance of the device the following should be high rather than low:

a. AC frequency of a diathermy (electrosurgical) unit.
b. Signal-to-noise ratio of ECG monitoring equipment.
c. Input impedance of an amplifier.
d. Electrical resistance in a mains earth cable.
e. Electrical impedance of antistatic footwear.

1.27 The following are true of the phenomenon of diamagnetism:

a. It is a property of all materials.
b. It is stronger than paramagnetism.
c. It is inversely related in strength to temperature.
d. Materials possessing the property have a relative permeability of less than unity.
e. Materials exhibiting it possess 'magnetic domains'.

1.28   The following relate to the activity of diathermy (electrosurgery):

a. Fulguration.
b. Interrogation current.
c. Cavitation.
d. Channelling.
e. Collimation.

1.29   In the case of CO_2 absorption by soda lime:

a. The chemical reaction is endothermic.
b. It is a reversible chemical reaction.
c. Water is essential for the reaction.
d. The reaction occurs better with cold than warm soda lime.
e. Water is a byproduct of the chemical reaction.

1.30   Antistatic precautions should be required in a modern operating theatre:

a. If explosive anaesthetic agents are being used.
b. If monopolar diathermy is being used.
c. If laser surgery is in progress.
d. To help minimize 'noise' at the contact points of ECG electrodes.
e. For the proper functioning of anaesthetic machine flowmeters.

1.31   The following statements are true:

a. The Seebeck effect refers to the electrical behaviour at the junction of two dissimilar metals.
b. The Poynting effect refers to the behaviour of a gas mixture inside a helium–oxygen cylinder.
c. The Joule–Thomson effect prevails when a gas is subjected to sudden severe compression.
d. The Raman effect is the scattering of a beam of monochromatic light when passed through a transparent medium, the scattered beam being at the same frequency as the incident beam.
e. The Doppler effect is the apparent change in the observed frequency of any type of wave as the result of relative motion between the source of the wave and the observer.

1.32   The following statements are true:

a. The higher the voltage of AC electricity the greater the energy losses during its transmission from the generator station to the consumer site.
b. The higher the frequency of AC electricity the greater the impedance to its passage through a capacitor.
c. The higher the frequency of electromagnetic radiations the greater their energy.
d. The higher the frequency of ultrasound waves the better the resolution of the images they produce.
e. The higher the input impedance of an ECG amplifier the greater the attenuation of the output ECG signal.

1.33   The following statements are true:

a. A perfect black body emitter reflects all radiant energy incident on it.
b. An ideal gas is one whose entities have perfectly elastic collisions with the bounding walls of their container.
c. A perfect solution is one that obeys Raoult's Law.
d. An ideal fluid is one whose viscosity remains constant despite change in its shear rate during flow.
e. A perfect capacitor in an AC circuit is regarded as having reactance but no resistance.

1.34   The following devices are examples of transducers:

a. The retina of the human eye.
b. A diagnostic ultrasound probe.
c. An X-ray tube.
d. A rectifier in an AC electrical circuit.
e. A mercury clinical thermometer.

1.35   The following properties of water are the result of hydrogen bonds present in it:

a. Polarity.
b. High dielectric constant.
c. High boiling point compared with most other common liquids.
d. High latent heat of vaporization.
e. A higher specific density than ice.

1.36   The following mean the same:

a. Zwitterion and ampholyte ion.
b. Amphipathicity and amphiphilicity.
c. Transition temperature and critical temperature.
d. Atomic mass unit and unified mass unit.
e. Atomic weight and dalton.

1.37   The following are or have been used as draw-over vaporizers:

a. EMO (Epstein–Macintosh–Oxford) vaporizer.
b. Goldman vaporizer.
c. Halox vaporizer.
d. Boyle 'bottle'.
e. Schimmelbusch mask.

1.38   The 'pumping effect' in relation to plenum vaporizers is likely to be less:

a. If the bypass chamber and vaporizing chamber are of equal volume.
b. If there is less liquid anaesthetic agent in the vaporizing chamber.
c. If the patient is on mechanical artificial ventilation rather than in spontaneous ventilation mode.
d. If a nonreturn valve is sited downstream of the vaporizer.
e. If there is a short gas inlet tube into the vaporizing chamber.

1.39 The following devices or systems, when operational, are subject to a pressure of the order of kilopascals rather than pascals:

a. 'Needle' valve at the base of the anaesthetic machine flowmeter tubes.
b. Oxygen cut-off warning device on the anaesthetic machine.
c. APL (adjustable pressure limiting) valve on a Magill breathing attachment (Mapleson A) during normal adult spontaneous ventilation.
d. Operating theatre plenum ventilation ('air-conditioning') system.
e. Gas flow through the vaporizing chamber of a Mark 4 plenum vaporizer.

1.40 The following symbols are correct:

a. 'Q' as an indicator of fluid flow rate.
b. 'R' as the indicator of electrical impedance.
c. 'KV' as an indicator of kilovolts.
d. 'gHz' as an indicator of gigahertz.
e. 'Pf' as an indicator of picoFarads.

1.41 Ultraviolet electromagnetic radiations are absorbed by:

a. Ozone.
b. Nitrous oxide.
c. Water vapour.
d. Halothane.
e. Helium.

1.42 White is the colour of whole or part of the shoulders of the following gas cylinders:

a. Oxygen.
b. Entonox.
c. Cyclopropane.
d. 5% CO_2 in oxygen.
e. Heliox (79% helium in oxygen).

1.43 The 'filling ratio' is applicable to cylinders containing the following:

a. Nitrogen.
b. Nitrous oxide.
c. Helium 79% in oxygen 21%.
d. Cyclopropane;
e. Air.

1.44 The amount of the agent contained in each of the following cylinders can only be determined by weighing the cylinder:

a. Oxygen cylinder.
b. Carbon dioxide cylinder.
c. 5% CO_2 in oxygen cylinder.
d. Entonox cylinder.
e. Nitrogen cylinder.

1.45   If an oxygen cylinder (on the anaesthetic machine) is 'bled' at a constant rate:

a. The pressure change shown on the cylinder gauge will give an accurate indication of the amount of oxygen remaining in the cylinder.
b. Frost is likely to form on the outside wall of the cylinder.
c. The cylinder contents are likely to show the Joule–Thomson effect.
d. The cylinder is likely to stop the escape of oxygen if water is a contaminant in it.
e. The internal energy change will be a conversion from kinetic to potential energy.

1.46   In the case of entonox cylinders:

a. They possess pin index outlets throughout the range of cylinder sizes.
b. Their largest size (which may be used for providing a piped supply) is size J.
c. Their size G cylinders can provide twice the volume of gas mixture (at 1 bar pressure) as size F cylinders.
d. They are subject to a filling ratio of 0.67 in the UK.
e. Their contents are prone to lamination on standing.

1.47   A gas pressure of about 4 bar is the norm in the following:

a. Air flow up an anaesthetic machine air flow rotameter tube.
b. Anaesthetic machine pressure relief valve at the downstream end of the back bar.
c. Pressure relief valve on an oxygen VIE (vacuum insulated evaporator).
d. Mains pipeline air drill for surgical purposes.
e. Pressure in mains entonox delivery pipelines.

1.48   Of the noble gases argon, helium, krypton, neon, radon and xenon:

a. Radon is the one in most abundance in the earth's atmosphere.
b. Helium is the lightest.
c. Neon has the lowest boiling point.
d. Krypton is the one by which the SI unit of length is now defined.
e. Xenon is the only one that possesses anaesthetic properties under normobaric conditions.

1.49   Helium:

a. Is used in laser surgery of the airways because it does not support combustion.
b. Could be useful in increasing heat loss via the respiratory tract.
c. Is a valuable substitute for nitrogen in hyperbaric applications.
d. Can cause voice distortion.
e. Is useful in upper airway obstruction because of its low viscosity.

1.50 The following phenomena are characteristic features of laser light energy:

a. Collimation.
b. Coherence.
c. Population inversion.
d. Remanence.
e. Cavitation.

1.1 Answers

a. True.
b. False – it is a *base* unit, not a fundamental unit.
c. False – the radian is a *supplementary* unit.
d. True.
e. False – it is the kilogram, not the gram, which is the fundamental unit.

Note: There are three fundamental units: metre, kilogram and second. The whole of mechanics can be dealt with using them in their dimensional format: (L), (M) and (T).

Note: Any physical equation, to be scientifically valid, must possess dimensional homogeneity, i.e. the dimensions on the two sides of the equation must be identical. Take the equation BP = CO × SVR:

Blood pressure = cardiac output × systemic vascular resistance

(force per unit area) = (flow rate) × (pressure per unit flow rate)

$$(M)\ (L)\ (T)^{-2}\ (L)^{-2} = (L)^3\ (T)^{-1} \times (M)\ (L)\ (T)^{-2}\ (L)^{-2} \times (L)^{-3}\ (T)$$

The units on the two sides of the equation are the same and therefore the equation is scientifically valid.

1.2 Answers

a. False – the siemens is the SI unit of electrical conductance (reciprocal of electrical resistance). Note its plural form, so the expression is '1 siemens', '2 siemens', etc. because it is named after Ernest Werner von Siemens (1816–1892). Its symbol is S and it was formerly called the mho or reciprocal ohm.

b. True – the stokes (symbol St) is the cgs unit of kinematic viscosity, and is the dynamic viscosity of a fluid (in poise) divided by its density. There is no named unit for kinematic viscosity in the SI nomenclature; 1 stokes = 10^{-4} m^2 s^{-1}. The kinematic viscosity is a factor in determining Reynolds number. Note again the plural form '1 stokes', as it is named after Sir George Gabriel Stokes (1819–1903).

c. False – the Gray (symbol Gy) is the derived SI unit of absorbed dose of ionizing radiation. It is a measure of the energy transferred to a substance by radiations and is equal to 1 J kg^{-1}. It is named after Louis Harold Gray (1905–1965), the radiobiologist.

d. True – symbol eV. A unit of energy (not voltage) equal to the work done in moving an electron through a potential difference of 1 V. 1 eV = 1.602×10^{-19} J.

e. True – the poise is the non-SI unit of dynamic viscosity, which in the SI nomenclature has no named unit and is expressed as newton seconds per metre^2 or pascal seconds.

1.3 Answers

a. True – because it does not possess any 'dimensions', i.e. (M), (L) or (T) in relation to the fundamental units. However, it is a 'unit' because it is the means of expressing the magnitude of the solid angle. But the solid angle (measured in steradians) and plane angle (measured in radians) are for some reason regarded as 'unitless'!

b. False – it, like the radian, is a *supplementary* unit.

c. False – see **a** above.

d. True – luminance (or photometric brightness) is the luminous intensity (arriving at a surface or leaving it or passing through it) in a given direction per unit projected area of the surface, viewed from that direction, and is measured in lumens per square metre per steradian (or candela per metre^2).

e. True – the lumen (symbol lm) is the SI unit of luminous flux equal to the flux emitted by a uniform point source of 1 cd in a solid angle of 1 steradian.

1.4 Answers

a. True – the unit is the ampere, which is the number of *coulombs per second* of electricity flowing in a circuit.

b. True – power is the rate of doing work and is measured in watts, i.e. joules per second.

c. True – it is the energy in the form of visible radiations (i.e. the light energy) reaching a surface of unit area in unit time, i.e. the luminous flux per unit time and is measured in lumens per square metre or lux.

d. False – although it is designated in pressure units per unit flow *rate* (e.g. centimetres water per litre per minute), it is not a rating.

e. False – capacitance is the ability of a system to store charge and is expressed in coulombs per volt.

1.5 Answers

a. False – ampere is a rating; it is coulombs per second; see **1.4a**.

b. False – the lumen is a 'power' unit, i.e. it is a measure of the flow of luminous energy.

c. False – watt is the unit of energy rating and is joules per second; see **1.4b**.

d. False – it is the unit of *dynamic* viscosity; see **1.2e**.

e. False – it is the unit of magnetic flux *density*; the unit of magnetic flux is the weber. Therefore 1 T = 1 Wb m^{-2}.

1.6   Answers

a. **True** – it is a ratio or a percentage: a measure of the extent by which the intensity of a light beam is reduced on passing through a distance d of a solution having a molar concentration m of the solute.

b. **True** – change of an electrical property (usually resistance with temperature) in relation to its previous value. Therefore it is a ratio and thus dimensionless.

c. **True** – the extent to which the oscillations in a vibrating system reduce in magnitude with each successive 'bounce'.

d. **False** – the diffusion coefficient is dependent on, among others, the Boltzmann constant, absolute temperature and viscosity of the medium.

e. **False** – it is the amount of a solute that passes through unit surface area (say of a capillary) per unit time per unit distance (of capillary wall thickness) and is expressed in moles per square centimetre per second per centimetre thickness, i.e. moles per centimetre per second.

1.7   Answers

a. **False** – the inverse square law applies to ordinary light because it diverges during transmission. Collimated light (such as that produced by a laser) does not diverge and therefore does not diminish in intensity with distance.

b. **True.**

c. **False** – the magnitude of van der Waals forces is inversely proportional to the seventh power of the distance separating them.

d. **False** – laminar flow is *directly* proportional the fourth power of the radius and therefore to the square of the cross-sectional area.

e. **False** – the total intensity of emitted radiations of a 'perfect black body' is *directly* proportional to the fourth power of its Kelvin temperature.

1.8   Answers

a. **True.**

b. **False** – the change is linear.

c. **False** – the change is linear.

d. **True.**

e. **True.**

1.9   Answers

a. **False** – the relationship is in accordance with the inverse square law: $A \propto 1/B^2$; see **5.9b**.

b. **True** – kinetic energy $= \frac{1}{2}mv^2$.

c. **True** – because energy in joules = voltage × current × time, but V is equal to current × resistance. Therefore energy = resistance × current^2 × time. Therefore energy $\propto$ current^2.

d. **False** – radiation energy $\propto T^4$, T being the Kelvin temperature.

e. **True** – the energy of EMRs is directly proportional to the square of the wave amplitude: $E \propto A^2$.

1.10 Answers

a. **False** – zero-order systems are 'linear' in their behaviour; time constants are a phenomenon of exponential systems, i.e. first-order systems.

b. **False** – it is longer than the half-life of a system. Half-life = 0.693 of the time constant.

c. **True.**

d. **True.**

e. **False** – it is equal to inductance divided by resistance.

1.11 Answers

a. **True.**

b. **True.**

c. **True.**

d. **True.**

e. **True** – the speed is directly proportional to the square root of its temperature.

1.12 Answers

a. **True** – adiabatic expansion, also known as the Joule–Kelvin effect because Sir William Thomson later became Lord Kelvin.

b. **True** – the validity of Boyle's Law is dependent on the conditions being isothermal, i.e. temperature is the constant and pressure and volume the variables.

c. **False.**

d. **True** – adiabatic expansion at the tip of the cryoprobe gives rise to the cooling effect.

e. **True** – adiabatic compression, if extreme, can cause a rise of temperature sufficient to cause a fire.

1.13 Answers

a. **True** – the shear stress on a Newtonian fluid (i.e. a fluid showing laminar flow), causing relative movement between the fluid layers, is equal to F/A, where F is the tangential force acting on the fluid and A is the area of each of the adjacent parallel layers of fluid.

b. **True** – Ohm's Law: $V = iR$; i.e. pressure = flow rate × resistance. Also compare blood pressure × cardiac output × systemic vascular resistance.

c. **False** – it is in accordance with the 'Square' Law, i.e. $A \propto B^2$. Note: the flow rate $\propto$ radius^4, which is the same as the square of the cross-sectional area.

d. **False** – density is an operational factor in turbulent flow.

e. **True** – because, by definition, a Newtonian fluid shows laminar flow, in which flow rate $\propto$ pressure gradient; see **b** above.

1.14 Answers

a. True – there is a slight Venturi effect at the patient end of the co-axial tube, when the gases from the inner (afferent) co-axial tube 'open out'and admix with gases in the outer (efferent) co-axial tube.

b. True.

c. True.

d. False – Pitot tube: a device for measuring speed of a fluid. It consists of two tubes, one whose opening faces the moving fluid and the other with an opening at 90° to the direction of flow. The two tubes are connected to the opposite ends of a manometer so that the difference in the dynamic pressure of the first tube and the static pressure in the second can be measured. The flow rate and therefore the total flow is proportional to the pressure difference.

e. True – when the oxygen (at 4 bar pressure) comes out of the needle attachment of the injector it entrains atmospheric air. So the patient is in effect ventilated with an oxygen-enriched supply of air.

1.15 Answers

a. True – volume expansion of mercury.

b. True – volume expansion of alcohol.

c. True – detects the differential expansion of the two metal strips.

d. False – measures a pressure change of a gas or vapour in accordance with Gay-Lussac's Law: the pressure of a fixed mass of gas of constant volume is directly related to its temperature.

e. False – by detecting a change in EMR frequency.

1.16 Answers

a. True.

b. False.

c. True.

d. True.

e. False.

1.17 Answers

a. False – volumes per cent.

b. True.

c. True.

d. True.

e. True.

1.18 Answers

a. True – mass spectrometry can measure any gas.

b. False – to be assayable by infrared analysis a gas must have at least two dissimilar atoms.

c. False.

d. True – a gas can be analysed by Raman scattering provided it is di-atomic, but the two atoms need not be different.

e. True.

1.19 Answers

a. **True** – therefore the presence of a 'rogue' gas vitiates the accuracy of the spectrometer.
b. **True.**
c. **True.**
d. **True.**
e. **False** – mass spectrometry can analyse any gas.

1.20 Answers

a. **True.**
b. **True.**
c. **True.**
d. **False** – N_2O is not a paramagnetic gas.
e. **False** – the method can analyse halogenated inhalational anaesthetic agents but not 'inorganic' gases such as O_2, N_2, N_2O and CO_2.

1.21 Answers

a. **True** – may underestimate the SpO_2 reading.
b. **True** – lowers readings in a dose-related manner.
c. **True** – lowers readings in a dose-related manner.
d. **True** – can lead to a lower reading.
e. **False.**

1.22 Answers

a. **True** – c. 80–100 mA.
b. **False** – of the order of amperes.
c. **True** – in DBS two short bursts of tetanus at 50 Hz at a supramaximal current of about 80 mA are applied to the nerve.
d. **True** – about 60 mA.
e. **False** – in the range of 1–2 A. The current has to be high because the resection is performed 'under water'.

1.23 Answers

a. **True** – as its name indicates, the platinum resistance thermometer detects a change in 'resistance', which is one form of impedance.
b. **True.**
c. **True** – it can do so by detecting changes in electrical resistance, capacitance or inductance, which are all forms of impedance.
d. **False** – the change detected is in voltage.
e. **False** – the change detected is one of potential difference.

1.24 Answers

a. False – a potential difference is only necessary if there is resistance to overcome in the circuitry. If the circuit is made of 'superconductor' material, as in the case of the electromagnet in an MRI scanner, no potential difference is necessary to make current flow. Compare Newton's First Law of Motion: a body continues in a state of uniform motion in a straight line unless it is acted upon by external forces. So, if there is no external force of friction (the corresponding property in an electrical circuit is impedance) it will continue to move at uniform speed; similarly, if there is no internal resistance to current flow then no potential difference is necessary for flow of current energy in an electrical circuit.

b. True – because voltage, current and resistance are related in accordance with Ohm's Law. So, the resistance being fixed, when the voltage varies, the current too varies in phase with it.

c. False – it is impedance that is the sum of reactance and resistance. Inductance is one form of reactance, the other being capacitance.

d. True – at resonant frequency the reactance of a capacitor and that of an inductor will cancel each other out, leaving resistance as the sole component of electrical impedance. Therefore, current will be maximal.

e. False – with direct current an energy level of about 20% greater than that with alternating current is required.

1.25 Answers

a. False – the standard discharge pattern is that of a 'damped sine wave', but more recent defibrillators have different wave forms: 'saw-toothed', 'rectilinear', etc. in both monophasic and biphasic forms.

b. True.

c. False – whether in 'cutting' mode or 'coagulating' mode the diathermy current is in the form of a sine wave.

d. True.

e. True.

1.26 Answers

a. True.

b. True.

c. True.

d. False – it should be as low as possible so as to maintain the defective equipment at near zero potential by conducting the leakage current as easily as possible to earth.

e. True – so as to allow ease of conduction of static electricity to earth but oppose that of mains electricity.

I.27 Answers

a. **True** – all substances are diamagnetic. It is a weak form of magnetism and may be masked by other, stronger, forms such as paramagnetism and ferromagnetism. It results from changes induced by the applied field in the orbits of electrons in the atoms of the substance. The direction of change is in accordance with Lenz's Law and therefore opposes the applied flux. There is thus a weak 'negative' susceptibility, i.e. the substance tends to move the magnetic field away from it.

b. **False** – it is weaker than paramagnetism.

c. **False** – it is unaffected by temperature.

d. **True** – just under I, because of the 'negative' susceptibility.

e. **False** – 'magnetic domains' are a feature of ferromagnetism.

I.28 Answers

a. **True** – fulguration (Latin: *fulgur*: lightning) refers to the use of high density diathermy current to excise tissues, the high density leading to lightning-like sparks ; hence the term fulguration.

b. **True** – an interrogation current checks the adequacy of apposition of an REM (return electrode monitoring) diathermy plate to the skin and thereby ensures that in the event of inadequate contact the definitive diathermy current does not flow, thus preventing a diathermy 'burn' of the skin under the plate.

c. **False** – cavitation is a phenomenon associated with ultrasound waves.

d. **True** – in channelling the (monopolar) diathermy current takes a return to the diathermy plate along attenuated tissue (such as a dissected and mobilized spermatic cord during an orchidopexy). The attenuated tissue would have a higher current density and this increases the risk of a rise in temperature in the tissue and consequential thermal damage (diathermy burn). Therefore bipolar diathermy is preferred in such situations.

e. **False** – collimation, nondivergence of a beam of radiant energy such as light, is a phenomenon of laser light.

I.29 Answers

a. **False** – it is an exothermic reaction; heat is produced in the process.

b. **False** – the reaction is irreversible.

c. **True** – see **e** below.

d. **False.**

e. **True** – the reaction takes place thus:
$$CO_2 + H_2O = H_2CO_3$$
$$NaOH + H_2CO_3 \rightarrow NaHCO_3 + H_2O$$
$$NaHCO_3 + Ca(OH)_2 \rightarrow CaCO_3 + NaOH + H_2O$$

I.30 Answers

a. **True.**

b. **False.**

c. **False.**

d. **True.**

e. **True.**

1.31 Answers

a. **True** – it is the change in potential (indicated by a voltage change).
b. **False** – it is the behaviour of the contents of an entonox cylinder.
c. **False** – it is the fall in temperature that results when there is sudden severe decompression of a gas.
d. **False** – at a different frequency, some at a higher, others at a lower frequency. Where the scattered light is at the same frequency it is known as Rayleigh scattering;
e. **True** – it applies to light waves as much as sound waves. In fact Doppler first noticed it with respect to light waves.

1.32 Answers

a. **False** – it is to reduce energy losses that mains electricity is transmitted at high voltages, between 125 000 and 400 000 V.
b. **False** – the impedance is less; cf. an inductor which has an impedance directly and linearly related to frequency.
c. **True** – the energy has a direct linear relationship with frequency via the equation: $E = h\,f$, where E is energy in joules, f is frequency in hertz, and h is the Planck constant, which has the value 6.626×10^{-34} J s.
d. **True** – but with higher frequency the penetrative ability of sound waves diminishes; hence the lower frequency of ships' foghorns which therefore increases the transmission of the audible warning they produce.
e. **False** – it improves the output signal.

1.33 Answers

a. **False** – a perfect black body emitter *absorbs* all radiations incident on it and *emits* all such radiations.
b. **True** – one of the definitional characteristics of an ideal gas.
c. **False** – it is an *ideal* solution that by definition obeys Raoult's Law. Raoult's Law generally only holds for dilute solutions. But where a solution obeys it over a whole range of concentrations it is called a *perfect* solution. So, although perfect solutions do conform to Raoult's Law, the definition of a 'perfect solution' is not one that obeys Raoult's Law.
d. **False** – an ideal fluid is one that is incompressible, i.e. it has no internal frictional forces viz. viscosity in it. It is a Newtonian fluid that has a constant viscosity despite a changing shear rate.
e. **False** – capacitors do not have *resistance*; they have *reactance*. A perfect capacitor has no reactance either.

1.34 Answers

a. **True** – converts light energy into an electrical signal.
b. **True** – converts electrical energy into sound energy and vice versa.
c. **True** – converts electrical energy into radiant energy.
d. **False** – a rectifier in an electrical circuit converts AC into DC.
e. **True** – converts heat energy into mechanical energy leading to expansion of the mercury.

1.35 Answers

a. **True.**
b. **True.**
c. **True.**
d. **True.**
e. **True.**

1.36 Answers

a. **True** – a substance that can act both as an acid as well as a base. Proteins are zwitterions and so is water because it can dissociate into H^+ (acid) and OH^- ions (base).
b. **True** – they refer to the ability of a structure to be both hydrophobic as well as hydrophilic. The cell wall is such a structure because of its phospholipid composition, the phospho part being hydrophilic and the lipid part being hydrophobic.
c. **True** – in the context of superconductivity. It is the temperature at which a conductor becomes superconductive. ('Critical temperature' also has another meaning: the temperature above which a gas cannot be liquefied by pressure alone.)
d. **True** – a unit of mass used to express relative atomic masses. It is 1/12th of the mass of an atom of the carbon-12 isotope and is equal to 1.66033×10^{-27} kg. It is also called the *dalton*.
e. **False** – the atomic weight, now known as the *relative atomic mass*, is the ratio of the average mass per atom of the naturally occurring form of the element to 1/12th the mass of a carbon-12 atom. Therefore it is a 'dimensionless entity'. The dalton (see **d** above) is a 'unitized' quantity.

1.37 Answers

a. **True.**
b. **True.**
c. **False.**
d. **False.**
e. **True.**

1.38 Answers

a. **False** – the vaporizing chamber should be of smaller volume.
b. **False** – if there is less liquid anaesthetic then there is a greater airspace above it which allows a greater pumping effect.
c. **False** – if there is mechanical artificial ventilation there is greater fluctuation of the back pressure on the flow of the anaesthetic gases and this leads to a greater pumping effect.
d. **True.**
e. **False** – a short gas inlet tube makes it easier for the 'back pressured' gases to enter the vaporizing chamber.

1.39 Answers

a. True – 400 kPa.

b. True – 400 kPa.

c. False – during normal spontaneous ventilation the APL valve is maintained in the 'full open' position, in which case the resistance to gas flow through it is of the order of less than 1 kPa per 7 L per minute gas flow rate.

d. False – the pressure gradient across the theatre is about 35 Pa.

e. True – the resistance to gas flow is c. 30 cmH_2O, i.e. c. 3 kPa.

1.40 Answers

a. False – the symbol is '$\dot{Q}$' i.e. Q with a dot on top of it.

b. False – although it is measured in ohms, impedance is denoted by 'Z'.

c. False – the notation is 'kV'.

d. False – the notation is 'GHz'.

e. False – the notation is 'pF'.

1.41 Answers

a. True.

b. False.

c. False.

d. True.

e. False.

1.42 Answers

a. True – wholly white, with a black body.

b. True – alternating white and blue quadrants, with a blue body.

c. False – a cyclopropane cylinder is orange throughout.

d. True – alternating white and grey quadrants with a black body.

e. True – white and brown alternating quadrants with a black body.

1.43 Answers

a. False.

b. True.

c. False.

d. True.

e. False.

1.44 Answers

a. False.

b. True.

c. False.

d. False.

e. False.

1.45 Answers

a. True – by application of the Universal Gas equation: $PV = nRT$.
b. False.
c. False.
d. False.
e. False – it is a change from potential to kinetic energy.

1.46 Answers

a. True.
b. False – the largest size is 'G'.
c. False – F cylinder: 2000 L; G cylinder: 5000 L.
d. False – since their contents are solely gaseous, 'filling ratio' does not apply.
e. True.

1.47 Answers

a. False – it is about 30–35 kPa.
b. False – about 35–40 kPa.
c. False – c. 7 bar.
d. False – c. 7 bar;
e. True – c. 4.1 bar.

1.48 Answers

a. False – argon: 0.93; radon: one part in 10^{21} parts of air.
b. True – because it has the lowest atomic weight of them all.
c. False – the boiling points (in Celsius) are: argon: −186; neon: −246; helium: −269; krypton: −52; radon: −62; xenon: −107.
d. False – it was so until 1983, but the metre is now defined with respect to the speed of light in a vacuum, i.e the distance travelled by light in 1/299 792 458th of a second.
e. True.

1.49 Answers

a. False – helium does not support combustion, but it is used in upper airway laser surgery because of its high thermal conductivity.
b. False – although it has a high thermal conductivity, helium is not useful in increasing heat loss via the respiratory tract because it is the *heat capacity* and not the *thermal conductivity* of the breathing mixture that is the relevant factor. The heat capacity of helium is less than that of air and therefore the agent is not of any use in increasing the respiratory component of heat loss.
c. True – the use of helium (with oxygen), rather than nitrogen, for diving activities is based on (a) its lack of narcotic potential even at high pressures, and (b) its relative insolubility in body tissues: solubility in water (volume of gas per unit volume of liquid) at 20 °C and one bar pressure: nitrogen: 0.02390; helium: 0.00912.
d. True – the high velocity of sound transmission in helium causes voice distortion.
e. False – because of its low density.

1.50 Answers

a. **True** – nondivergence of light beam. Therefore, laser light does not obey the inverse square law.

b. **True** – i.e. all the waves are in phase.

c. **True** – the presence of a higher percentage of energized electrons in the electron population compared with the quiescent electrons, i.e. those in the resting state.

d. **False** – remanence is a property of ferromagnetism. It refers to the presence of some residual magnetic flux density in a ferromagnetic substance even after the saturating field has returned to zero.

e. **False** – cavitation is a phenomenon of ultrasound: the expansion of microbubbles in a liquid or near-liquid medium as a result of US energy. If they did so to the point of very sudden collapse an enormous rise of temperature could occur with consequent severe tissue damage.

Practice paper 2

2.1 The following are non-SI units:

    a. Centimetre water (as a unit of pressure measurement).
    b. Electron-volt.
    c. Calorie.
    d. Bar.
    e. Decilitre.

2.2 The following are 'derived' units under the SI units system:

    a. Pascal.
    b. Curie.
    c. Steradian.
    d. Angstrom.
    e. Siemens.

2.3 The following 'quantities' express 'intensity,' i.e. they may correctly be regarded as expressing the manifestation of a phenomenon in relation to unit surface area:

    a. Surface tension.
    b. Stress.
    c. Strain.
    d. Weight.
    e. Density.

2.4 The following units of pressure are independent of changes in gravity:

    a. Newtons per square metre.
    b. Pounds per square inch.
    c. Dynes per square centimetre.
    d. Centimetres water pressure.
    e. Torr.

2.5 The following statements are true:

    a. The unit of electrical capacitance is the coulomb.
    b. The unit of electrical inductance is the weber.
    c. The unit of magnetic flux is the tesla.
    d. The unit of electrical impedance is the ohm.
    e. The unit of electrical reactance is the siemens.

2.6 The following equations in physics are correct:

    a. Watts $\times$ seconds = joules.
    b. Coulombs $\times$ seconds = amperes.
    c. Lumens $\times$ seconds = talbots.
    d. Amperes $\times$ ohms^2 = joules.
    e. Pressure $\times$ volume = work done.

2.7　The following are 'dimensionless entities':

a. Diffusion coefficient.
b. Oil–gas partition coefficient.
c. Temperature coefficient.
d. Sieving coefficient.
e. Osmotic coefficient.

2.8　The following pairs of quantities have the same units:

a. Surface tension and pressure.
b. Electrical impedance and electrical reactance.
c. Intensity of illumination ('brightness') and luminous flux.
d. Stress and strain.
e. Electrical conductance and electrical capacitance.

2.9　The following relationships when graphically represented take the form of an accelerating growth exponential:

a. Pressure and volume of an ideal gas in accordance with Boyle's Law.
b. Specific density of 'physiological' urine and its osmolarity.
c. The electrical resistance of a metal conductor and its temperature.
d. Flow rate and pressure in the case of turbulent flow of a fluid.
e. Intra-alveolar pressure change during the inspiratory phase of IPPV with a constant pressure generator ventilator.

2.10　The following have the mathematical relationship $A \propto B^2$:

a. Light intensity and the amplitude of light waves.
b. In laminar flow, the flow rate and the cross-sectional area of the conduit.
c. The molecular weight of a substance and its rate of passive diffusion down its concentration gradient.
d. The total energy emitted per second by a perfect black body radiator and its Kelvin temperature.
e. The electrical energy in a system and the current flowing in it.

2.11　The following statements are true:

a. Laminar flow of fluid in a tube has a parabolic front.
b. The change in intra-alveolar pressure during the inspiratory phase of IPPV with a constant flow generator ventilator is exponential in nature.
c. The relationship between the threshold current for inducing VF and the frequency of that (alternating) current approximates to that of a hyperbola.
d. The temperature display curve in the case of a thermistor measuring device exhibits hysteresis.
e. The relationship between haematocrit and blood viscosity is linear.

2.12   **Adiabatic expansion of a gas:**

a. Can occur at the Bodok seal junction on an anaesthetic machine.
b. Will negate Boyle's Law in relation to the behaviour of a gas.
c. Occurs during the fractional distillation of air.
d. Occurs during conversion of liquid oxygen to gaseous oxygen in a vacuum-insulated evaporator.
e. Involves overcoming van der Waals forces of attraction between gas molecules.

2.13   **When there is turbulent flow in a fluid system:**

a. Flow rate has a direct linear relationship to pressure gradient.
b. Reynolds number for the system is less than 2000.
c. The flow is akin to that in the lower airways during normal quiet breathing.
d. The flow front has a parabolic profile.
e. The viscosity of the flowing fluid is a material factor in determining flow rate.

2.14   **An 'ideal solution':**

a. Is the same as a 'perfect solution'.
b. Is by definition one that is incompressible.
c. Has a relationship between osmotic pressure, volume and temperature in the same way as an ideal gas does in the Universal Gas equation.
d. Conforms to the van't Hoff's equation.
e. Conforms to Raoult's Law.

2.15   **The following are correct descriptions of 'critical temperature':**

a. The temperature above which a gas cannot be liquefied by pressure alone.
b. The temperature at which a liquid spontaneously changes into a gas, i.e. without the need for additional heat energy (latent heat of vaporization).
c. The temperature at which a conductor acquires the property of 'superconductivity'.
d. The temperature at which a gas most closely approximates to an ideal gas.
e. The temperature above which a material loses its ferromagnetism.

2.16   **Xenon:**

a. Is the only noble gas that can be used as a general anaesthetic under normobaric conditions.
b. Has a higher MAC value than nitrous oxide.
c. Exerts an analgesic effect via $\alpha 2$ and opioid receptors.
d. Enhances catecholamine release from surgical stimulation.
e. Is found in air at a higher concentration than argon.

2.17 The following are attributes of the phenomenon of ferromagnetism:

a. Presence of 'magnetic domains'.
b. It is unaffected by temperature.
c. Its materials have a relative permeability very near unity.
d. Its materials show hysteresis with respect to magnetization and demagnetization.
e. Remanence.

2.18 The following devices when operational have a voltage of about 5000 V:

a. Diathermy (electrosurgical) unit.
b. DC defibrillator.
c. MRI scanner.
d. CO_2 laser machine.
e. US scanner.

2.19 In the case of electromagnetic radiations (EMRs):

a. They all travel at the speed of light.
b. They only exist at temperatures above 0 kelvin.
c. Their plane of propagation is at right angles to their amplitude.
d. They are more likely to be mutagenic the longer their wavelengths.
e. They are visible in the 'infrared' range.

2.20 In the case of the bipolar mode of surgical diathermy:

a. Its use does not require a diathermy (return electrode) plate.
b. It necessitates the use of a hand-held switch.
c. It is the better diathermy mode for 'cutting'.
d. It minimizes the risk of 'channelling'.
e. It is the preferred mode for transurethral electrosurgical ablation (TUR) of the prostate gland.

2.21 The following refer to the same thing:

a. Magnetic field strength and magnetic flux.
b. 'Isolated' patient electrical circuit and 'floating' circuit.
c. 'Diathermy' and 'cautery'.
d. 'Class II' electrical equipment and 'doubly insulated' electrical equipment.
e. 'Reactance' in an electrical circuit and 'impedance' in an electrical circuit.

2.22 In the case of electrical cardioconversion of VF:

a. The determinant electrical parameter is voltage.
b. Other things being equal, DC electricity is more effective than AC electricity.
c. Biphasic energy wave forms have a higher safety margin than monophasic waveforms.
d. The current required is of the order of milliamperes.
e. The only dynamic impedance to the delivery of electricity to the heart is that presented by the patient's chest wall.

2.23   The following are examples of transducers:

  a. An incandescent electric light bulb.
  b. The 'phosphor' of a fluorescent 'strip' light.
  c. A sound microphone.
  d. A von Recklinghausen oscillotonometer used for measuring blood pressure.
  e. The capacitor in a DC defibrillator.

2.24   The risk of electrocution by electrical appliances is decreased if the:

  a. Equipment is of Class I type rather than Class II type.
  b. Casing of the appliance is at 'near zero potential'.
  c. Equipment has low amplifier input impedance.
  d. Equipment has a high 'signal-to-noise' ratio.
  e. Handler of the equipment has a high skin impedance.

2.25   An electrical capacitor can correctly be a component part of:

  a. A diathermy (electrosurgical) unit.
  b. A DC defibrillator.
  c. An electrical transformer.
  d. A fluid-coupled transducer for invasive arterial blood pressure measurement.
  e. A light emitting diode.

2.26   The risks of ventricular fibrillation are increased:

  a. With increasing frequency of alternating electric current.
  b. If the current is of the order of amperes rather than milliamperes.
  c. For the same current energy if the current is DC rather than AC.
  d. If the subject is using SELV equipment rather than Class I equipment.
  e. If the defective equipment is 'earthed' rather than 'non-earthed'.

2.27   A high electrical 'current density' is a desirable feature for the proper working of the following:

  a. Water heating in an electric kettle.
  b. Lighting up of an incandescent electric light bulb.
  c. Satisfactory working of a surgical diathermy forceps.
  d. Safe conductance of electricity via a diathermy plate.
  e. Conduction of an ECG signal through an ECG electrode.

2.28   A relative humidity of 40–60% of the theatre environment is advisable:

  a. For the physical comfort of theatre staff.
  b. If explosive anaesthetic agents are being used.
  c. To prevent build up of static electricity.
  d. To effectively minimize body heat loss from the patient.
  e. To render safe the use of diathermy (electrosurgery).

2.29   The following statements are true:

   a. The lower the temperature of a medium, the faster the speed of propagation of light through it.
   b. The lower the strength of an acid, the better its buffering ability.
   c. The lower the cardiac output of a patient, the more rapid the rate of inhalational induction.
   d. The lower the degree of ionization of an agent in the renal tubular fluid, the faster its rate of elimination in the urine.
   e. The lower the blood gas partition coefficient of an inhalational anaesthetic agent, the faster the rate of anaesthetic induction.

2.30   Other things being equal, the output concentration of an anaesthetic vaporizer is initially increased if the following are higher rather than lower:

   a. Density of carrier gases.
   b. Viscosity of carrier gases.
   c. Solubility of carrier gases in liquid anaesthetic agent.
   d. Temperature of the vaporizer chamber.
   e. Fresh gas flow rate.

2.31   The 'pumping effect' in respect of anaesthetic vaporizers can be reduced by:

   a. Reducing the capacity of the liquid chamber.
   b. Having a shorter gas inlet tube into the vaporizer chamber.
   c. Minimizing rapid fall in pressure during the expiratory phase.
   d. Having a smaller volume of liquid anaesthetic agent in the vaporizing chamber.
   e. Siting a one-way check valve at the common gas outlet.

2.32   A constant flow generator ventilator:

   a. Shows a progressively diminishing pressure differential between ventilator bellows and lungs during the inspiratory phase.
   b. Normally effects active gas elimination from the lungs during the expiratory phase.
   c. Can logically be a 'minute volume divider' ventilator.
   d. Must necessarily be energized by pressurized gases.
   e. Is exemplified by the Penlon AV 900 ventilator.

2.33   The Waters to-and-fro anaesthetic breathing attachment:

   a. Is a Mapleson C attachment.
   b. Can be modified to act as a Mapleson A attachment.
   c. When used for spontaneous ventilation with a fresh gas flow comparable with patient minute volume contains solely fresh gases in the breathing bag'.
   d. Can be suitably adapted as a low flow breathing attachment.
   e. Can if down-sized be used safely for paediatric ventilation.

2.34 **The following pairs bear an inverse relationship to each other:**

   a. The blood gas partition coefficient of an inhalational anaesthetic agent and its MAC value.
   b. The degree of dissociation of a substance in gastric juice and its rate of absorption through the gastric mucosa.
   c. The degree of dissociation of a drug in renal tubular fluid and its rate of renal elimination.
   d. The density of a medium and the speed of sound waves in it.
   e. The thickness of the dielectric of a capacitor and the capacitance of the capacitor.

2.35 **Halothane can be assayed by the following methods of gas analysis:**

   a. Mass spectrometry.
   b. Raman scattering.
   c. Ultraviolet gas analysis.
   d. Paramagnetic analysis.
   e. Piezo-electric method of gas analysis.

2.36 **The following gases can be assayed by infrared analysis:**

   a. Xenon.
   b. Oxygen.
   c. Nitrogen.
   d. Carbon monoxide.
   e. Nitrogen dioxide.

2.37 **Capnography by infrared analysis:**

   a. Is based on the principle enshrined in the Beer–Lambert Law.
   b. Is a rapid and reliable indicator of oesophageal intubation.
   c. Is a reliable pointer to endobronchial intubation.
   d. Can be vitiated by the presence of nitrous oxide in the gas sample.
   e. Can be adversely affected by the presence of glass windows in the analysing chamber.

2.38 **The 20 or so common amino acids in the body:**

   a. Are all α amino acids.
   b. Are all chiral.
   c. Are all of the L configuration.
   d. Are all S as opposed to R amino acids.
   e. Are all aliphatic amino acids.

2.39 **The following refer to the same thing:**

   a. Avogadro's number and Avogadro's constant.
   b. Amphipathicity and amphibolicity.
   c. Amphotericity and amphiphilicity.
   d. Electrical impedance and electrical resistance.
   e. A 'normal' solution and a 'molar' solution.

2.40   The Venturi effect:

a. Is based on the principle of the law of conservation of mechanical energy.
b. Applies to the flow of gases as well as liquids in tubes.
c. Is the result of conversion of kinetic energy into potential energy.
d. Is the basis of operation of a fixed performance oxygen mask.
e. Has been applied in the performance of suction apparatus.

2.41   The following are measured in decibels:

a. Intensity of sound.
b. Strength of a seismic wave (earthquake).
c. 'Signal-to-noise ratio' of monitoring equipment.
d. 'Gain' of an amplifier.
e. Common mode rejection ratio of monitoring equipment.

2.42   The following assertions are correct:

a. Relative humidity can be expressed as:

$$\frac{\text{actual mass of water vapour in the atmosphere}}{\text{maximum mass the atmosphere can hold}}$$

as well as:

$$\frac{\text{actual vapour pressure}}{\text{saturation vapour pressure.}}$$

b. Surface tension can be expressed as: newtons per metre as well as joules per square metre.
c. Avogadro's constant can be expressed both as the number of molecules of a gas in 1 gram mole and number of atoms of a gas in 1 gram mole.
d. The boiling point of a liquid can be expressed as the temperature at which the agent boils and the temperature at which the saturation vapour pressure of the agent equals atmospheric pressure.
e. Both electrical impedance and electrical resistance can be expressed in the unit of ohms.

2.43   The Bourdon gauge as a measure of pressure to indicate the amount of a cylinder contents is useful with respect to gas pressures in cylinders containing the following:

a. Carbon dioxide.
b. Entonox.
c. Cyclopropane.
d. 20% oxygen in 80% helium.
e. 5% CO_2 in oxygen.

2.44   The following gases have a critical temperature above 0 °C:

a. Helium.
b. Nitrogen.
c. Carbon dioxide.
d. Ethylene oxide.
e. Xenon.

2.45 The following cylinders, on an anaesthetic machine, necessarily need a pressure regulator in the gas pathway between the cylinder and the flowmeter unit:

a. Oxygen.
b. Nitrous oxide.
c. Carbon dioxide.
d. Cyclopropane.
e. Air.

2.46 Grey is part or whole of the colour of the shoulders of the following gas cylinders:

a. Oxygen.
b. Carbon dioxide.
c. 5% CO_2 in oxygen.
d. Air.
e. Nitrogen.

2.47 An oxygen cylinder:

a. Should have a filling ratio of 0.67 in the UK.
b. Has a colour coding for UK cylinders which includes a white and grey shoulder.
c. Needs to have been stored upright immediately prior to use.
d. Must be maintained upright when in use.
e. When full has a pressure of 137 bar, no matter the size of cylinder.

2.48 A size E oxygen cylinder:

a. When full has the same pressure as a size G oxygen cylinder.
b. Contains twice the amount of oxygen as a size D cylinder.
c. Has an empty weight approximately half that of a size F oxygen cylinder.
d. Is normally available with a pin index head.
e. Can be connected to an anaesthetic machine.

2.49 With regard to nitrous oxide cylinders:

a. J cylinders are the norm for a cylinder bank.
b. An F cylinder can be attached to the modern day anaesthetic machine.
c. An E cylinder has twice as much nitrous oxide as an F cylinder.
d. A Bourdon gauge is a useful indicator of the amount of agent in them.
e. A pressure regulator is an essential requirement in their gas pathway in an anaesthetic machine.

2.50 The following relate to the behaviour of laser light:

a. Stimulated emission.
b. Population inversion.
c. Remanence.
d. Gyromagnetic ratio.
e. Graded-index fibre.

2.1 Answers

a. **True.**
b. **True.**
c. **True.**
d. **True.**
e. **True.**

2.2 Answers

a. **True.**
b. **False** – the curie is not an SI unit; its corresponding SI unit is the becquerel.
c. **False** – the steradian is one of the two *supplementary* units in the SI system, the other being the radian.
d. **False.**
e. **True** – the siemens is the unit of electrical conductance, formerly called the mho or the reciprocal ohm.

2.3 Answers

a. **True** – surface tension is normally expressed in newtons per *metre*. This is the same as joules per *square metre*, which is the energy per unit surface area required to maintain the integrity of a liquid surface.
b. **True** – stress has the same units as pressure, i.e. newtons per square metre.
c. **False** – strain is a ratio and therefore is a 'dimensionless entity'.
d. **False** – weight is the force of gravity acting on a body and is equal to mass × acceleration due to gravity (the latter is now called 'acceleration of free fall').
e. **False** – density is a quantity related to unit *volume*.

2.4 Answers

a. **True** – one of the prerequisites of an SI unit is that it shall be independent of the effects of gravity.
b. **False.**
c. **True.**
d. **False.**
e. **False.**

2.5 Answers

a. **False** – the coulomb is the unit of charge or quantity of electricity. The unit of capacitance is the farad.
b. **False** – the weber is the unit of magnetic flux. The unit of electrical inductance is the henry, which is the inductance of a closed electrical circuit in which an EMF of 1 V is produced when the current in the circuit varies uniformly at a rate of 1 A s^{-1}.
c. **False** – the unit of magnetic flux is the weber. It is the magnetic flux equal to the flux that, linking a circuit of one turn, produces in it an EMF of 1 V as it is reduced to 0 at a uniform rate in 1 s. The tesla is the unit of magnetic flux density, i.e. webers per square metre.
d. **True.**
e. **False** – the siemens is the unit of electrical conductance. The unit of electrical reactance is the ohm.

2.6 Answers

a. **True.**
b. **False** – amperes × seconds = coulombs.
c. **True.**
d. **False** – ohms × amperes^2 × seconds = joules.
e. **True.**

2.7 Answers

a. **False** – the diffusion coefficient for a membrane is the total permeability of the membrane, i.e. the permeability × area of membrane: D × P × A, where permeability expresses movement of a substance through *unit* membrane area.
b. **True** – the oil–gas partition coefficient is the ratio in which an agent, at equilibrium, distributes itself between two compartments of equal volume of oil and gas separated by a membrane which is freely permeant to the agent.
c. **True** – the temperature coefficient is a coefficient that quantifies the degree of change of some physical property (e.g. electrical resistance) with change in temperature.
d. **True** – the sieving coefficient of a solute is the ratio of the concentration of that solute in the glomerular ultrafiltrate to its concentration in the plasma.
e. **True** – the osmotic coefficient is a measure of the extent to which an electrolyte dissociates. If there is 100% dissociation the osmotic coefficient is 1.

2.8 Answers

a. **False** – surface tension: newtons per metre or joules per square metre; pressure: newtons per square metre.
b. **True** – the unit is the ohm.
c. **False** – intensity of illumination (a base quantity in the SI system): candela; luminous flux (rate of flow of luminous energy emitted from a light source): lumen.
d. **False** – stress has the same units as pressure; strain is a ratio and therefore a dimensionless entity.
e. **False** – electrical conductance (the opposite of resistance): siemens; electrical capacitance: farad.

2.9 Answers

a. **False** – the relationship is inverse and therefore the graph is a rectangular hyperbola.
b. **False** – the change is virtually linear; if the urine were 'unphysiological', i.e. it had protein, then the relationship could be one of an accelerating growth exponential.
c. **False** – it is linear.
d. **True** – pressure on the y axis and flow on the x axis.
e. **False** – it is a decelerating growth exponential.

2.10 Answers

a. **True** – the energy of EMRs is proportional to the square of the amplitude of the waves.

b. **True** – flow rate $\propto$ radius^4; which is equivalent to cross-sectional area^2.

c. **False** – the flow rate is inversely proportional to the square root of the molecular weight (Graham's Law): $D \propto \dfrac{1}{\sqrt{MW}}$.

d. **False** – the energy is proportional to the fourth power of the Kelvin temperature: $E \propto T^4$;

e. **True** – energy (in joules) $\propto$ current^2.

2.11 Answers

a. **True.**

b. **False** – it is linear.

c. **True.**

d. **True.**

e. **False** – it is an accelerating growth exponential (viscosity on y axis, haematocrit on x axis).

2.12 Answers

a. **False** – it is adiabatic compression that is likely to occur.

b. **True** – in Boyle's Law temperature is the constant.

c. **True.**

d. **True.**

e. **True** – this is what consumes energy, resulting in the fall in temperature.

2.13 Answers

a. **False** – flow rate is proportional to the square root of the pressure gradient: $F \propto \sqrt{P}$.

b. **False** – it is more than 2000.

c. **False** – it is akin to that at the glottis.

d. **False** – it has a 'truncated' front.

e. **False** – it is density that is a material factor.

2.14 Answers

a. **False** – an ideal solution is, by definition, one that conforms to Raoult's Law; see **e** below. Only dilute solutions obey Raoult's Law, but if a solution obeys Raoult's Law over a greater range of concentrations it is called a perfect solution.

b. **False** – it is an ideal liquid that is incompressible.

c. **True** – π (osmotic pressure) = ρRT, where ρ is density, i.e. n/V (number of moles per unit volume). This is the same as the Universal Gas equation $PV = nRT$, i.e. $P = \dfrac{n}{V} RT$.

d. **True** – π (osmotic pressure) = ρRT is the van't Hoff equation.

e. **True** – see **a** above. Raoult's Law: the partial vapour pressure of a solvent is proportional to its mole fraction. If p is the vapour pressure of a solvent containing a substance in it and X the mole fraction of the solvent, then $p = p_o X$, where p_o is the vapour pressure of the pure solvent.

2.15 Answers

a. True.
b. True.
c. True – also known as the transition temperature.
d. False – this is known as the Boyle temperature.
e. False – this is known as the Curie temperature.

2.16 Answers

a. True.
b. False – lower MAC value; xenon: 0.71; N_2O: 1.05.
c. True.
d. False.
e. False – argon: 0.93%; xenon: 0.00087%.

2.17 Answers

a. True.
b. False – on heating it to its *Curie temperature* a ferromagnetic material loses its ferromagnetic property.
c. False – the relative permeability is very high;
d. True.
e. True – *remanence*: the amount of *magnetic intensity* left in a ferromagnetic core when the *magnetizing force* has declined to zero.

2.18 Answers

a. True.
b. True.
c. False.
d. False.
e. False.

2.19 Answers

a. True.
b. True.
c. True – contrast sound waves which have an amplitude in the same plane as their plane of propagation.
d. False – the shorter their wavelengths, the higher their possible mutagenicity.
e. False – the visible range ('light') is c. 380 nm (wavelength) for violet to c. 680 nm for red. Therefore 'infrared' is outside the visible range.

2.20 Answers

a. True.
b. False – it can be operated with a foot switch.
c. False – monopolar diathermy is the established mode for cutting;
d. True.
e. False – monopolar diathermy is the preferred mode.

2.21 Answers

a. False – magnetic flux (symbol φ) is a measure of the quantity of magnetism, taking account of the strength and extent of a magnetic field.

b. True – the circuit is 'earth-free'.

c. False – in diathermy some part of the patient tissue forms part of the electrical circuit. In 'cautery' heat produced in an electrical circuit is applied to the patient's tissue, which does not form part of the circuit, i.e. the conduction pathway. Indeed, there may not be any use of electricity at all, and heat may not be the energy form for cauterization; chemical cautery alone might do, e.g. use of $AgNO_3$ sticks for nasal cautery.

d. True.

e. False – reactance is only one form of impedance, the other being resistance.

2.22 Answers

a. False – the determinant electrical parameter is current energy (joules).

b. True.

c. True.

d. False – of the order of 20–30 A.

e. False – there is also the dynamic impedance of the electrical circuitry.

2.23 Answers

a. True – converts electrical energy to light energy.

b. False – the phosphor merely changes the frequencies of the EMRs to ones that are in the visible range.

c. True – converts sound energy to electrical energy.

d. False.

e. False.

2.24 Answers

a. False – although Class I equipment has an earth cable, Class II equipment is 'double insulated'.

b. True – this is the feature of Class I equipment.

c. False – low amplifier input affects the fidelity of production of the signal.

d. False – the signal-to-noise ratio has no bearing on the safety of equipment; like input impedance, it relates to the accuracy of equipment.

e. True – because it will reduce the amount of current passing through the person, perhaps to just a few milliamperes.

2.25 Answers

a. **True** – the purpose of the capacitor is to ensure that no electricity flows in the diathermy circuit if its frequency is below a critical level.

b. **True** – it is a necessary device; it stores the current energy and has it ready available for cardioconversion.

c. **False.**

d. **True** – the transducer changes mechanical energy (the force of the oscillating fluid) to electrical energy, which can be quantified as a change in resistance, inductance or capacitance; hence the possible presence of a capacitor in the measuring system.

e. **False.**

2.26 Answers

a. **False** – they are decreased; hence the use of high frequency current for diathermy.

b. **False** – at the order of amperes, electric current is more likely to cause cardiac standstill than VF.

c. **False** – as a general rule DC electricity needs to be about 20% greater in quantity than AC to produce VF.

d. **False** – SELV: safety extra low voltage.

e. **False** – if there is a properly connected and functioning earth cable, in the case of a leakage current the equipment would be at 'near zero potential' and therefore less likely to cause the passage of the leakage current through the subject.

2.27 Answers

a. **True.**

b. **True.**

c. **True.**

d. **False** – a low current density is required to obviate the risk of a diathermy burn of the skin under the diathermy plate.

e. **False** – it will attenuate the signal.

2.28 Answers

a. **True.**

b. **True** – because this will help reduce the build up of static electricity.

c. **True.**

d. **False** – the relative humidity level of 40–60% is insufficient to minimize body heat loss.

e. **False.**

2.29 Answers

a. **False** – the speed of light is not affected by the temperature of the medium of propagation.

b. **True** – a buffer is a *weak* acid and its conjugate base (or a weak base and its conjugate acid).

c. **True** – a decrease in cardiac output will increase the F_A/F_I ratio and thereby enhance the uptake of anaesthetic agents. But this only applies to highly soluble agents. Poorly soluble agents do not show significant change in the rate of uptake.

d. **False** – the higher the degree of ionization the less the tubular re-absorption and therefore the faster the rate of renal elimination.

e. **True.**

2.30 Answers

a. **True** – an increase in density of a carrier gas augments flow through the vaporizing chamber with a consequent small increase in agent output.

b. **True.**

c. **False.**

d. **True.**

e. **False.**

2.31 Answers

a. **True.**

b. **False.**

c. **True.**

d. **False** – if there is a smaller volume of liquid agent, there will be a greater air space above it. This will allow for more volume of volatilized agent, which will enhance the pumping effect.

e. **True.**

2.32 Answers

a. **False** – to maintain a constant flow rate during the inspiratory phase there has to be a constant pressure differential between ventilator bellows and lungs.

b. **False** – all ventilators, no matter their type, normally effect gas elimination by a passive process viz. the elastic recoil of the lungs.

c. **True** – by definition, in the case of a 'minute volume divider' only one of the parameters, tidal volume or ventilation rate, can be pre-set. In the case of a constant flow generator ventilator the tidal volume and ventilation rate (the two parameters that determine minute volume) are independently pre-set. But there is no logical reason why they cannot be determined by 'minute volume division'.

d. **False** – the ventilator can be energized by electricity as for instance in the case of the now obsolete Cape Waine ventilator.

e. **True.**

2.33 Answers

    a. True.
    b. False – Mapleson A is the Magill attachment.
    c. False – a mixture of fresh and exhaled gases.
    d. True – by incorporating a soda lime canister between the APL valve and breathing bag.
    e. False – not in its present form because of the presence of a spring-loaded APL valve, as valves are not permitted in paediatric breathing attachments because of the increased resistance they create during expiration. But it has been so used in the past.

2.34 Answers

    a. False – the blood gas partition coefficient is inversely related to the speed of induction, not to the potency of the agent. The latter is dependent on the fat–blood partition coefficient.
    b. True.
    c. False – it is a direct relationship; see **2.29d**.
    d. False – the denser the medium the faster the speed of sound.
    e. True – capacitance = $\varepsilon \times \dfrac{A}{d}$, where ε is the permittivity of the dielectric, A is the area of overlap of capacitance plates and d is the thickness of the dielectric.

2.35 Answers

    a. True.
    b. True.
    c. True – halothane vapour shows a strong absorption for ultraviolet light at about 200 nm.
    d. False.
    e. True.

2.36 Answers

    a. False.
    b. False.
    c. False.
    d. True.
    e. True.

2.37 Answers

    a. True.
    b. True.
    c. False.
    d. True.
    e. True – therefore the windows are made of sapphire.

2.38 Answers

    a. True – the amino ($-NH_2$) group is attached to the α carbon atom.
    b. False – the first amino acid – glycine – is achiral.
    c. True.
    d. False.
    e. False.

2.39 Answers

a. **True** – is the number of atoms in 1 mole: $6.022 \times 10^{23}\,mol^{-1}$.

b. **False** – amphipathicity is the property of being both hydrophilic and hydrophobic. The cell wall is amphipathic. Amphibolicity is the ability of a series of reactions in a biochemical pathway to take place in both directions. The Krebs cycle is an amphibolic pathway.

c. **True** – ability to act as an acid as well as an alkali, depending on the environmental pH.

d. **False** – impedance is a generic term to denote the opposition to current flow in an AC circuit which has both resistance and reactance. So resistance is only one form of impedance.

e. **False** – a normal solution contains 1 g equivalent of the solute per litre of solution. A molar solution contains 1 g mol of solute L^{-1} of solution.

2.40 Answers

a. **True.**

b. **True.**

c. **False** – the energy conversion is from potential to kinetic.

d. **True.**

e. **True** – a suction apparatus may be operated by the passage of pressurized gas (usually oxygen) through a Venturi device.

2.41 Answers

a. **True.**

b. **False** – this is measured on the Richter scale.

c. **True.**

d. **False.**

e. **False.**

2.42 Answers

a. **True.**

b. **True.**

c. **False** – this is only possible in the case of a monoatomic gas (such as helium).

d. **True.**

e. **True.**

2.43 Answers

a. **False.**

b. **True.**

c. **False.**

d. **True.**

e. **True.**

2.44 Answers

a. **False** – –267 °C.

b. **False** – –147 °C.

c. **True** – 31 °C.

d. **True** – 196 °C.

e. **True** – 16.5 °C.

2.45 Answers

a. **True.**
b. **True.**
c. **True.**
d. **False** – a full cyclopropane cylinder is at a pressure of only 7 bar.
e. **True.**

2.46 Answers

a. **False** – the shoulder is entirely white.
b. **True** – wholly grey, as is the body of the cylinder.
c. **True** – alternating grey and white quadrants.
d. **False** – the shoulder is of alternating black and white quadrants. The body is grey.
e. **False.**

2.47 Answers

a. **False** – filling ratios do not apply to oxygen cylinders because their contents are always entirely gaseous.
b. **False** – white shoulders.
c. **False.**
d. **False** – need not be because the contents are solely gaseous.
e. **True.**

2.48 Answers

a. **True** – see **e** above.
b. **True** – D cylinder 340 L; E cylinder 680 L.
c. **False** – E cylinder: 5.4 kg; F cylinder: 14.5 kg.
d. **True.**
e. **True** – it is the standard size for an anaesthetic machine.

2.49 Answers

a. **False** – nitrous oxide cylinders, unlike oxygen cylinders, stop at size G.
b. **False** – size E is the largest that can be attached to an anaesthetic machine.
c. **True** – E cylinder: 1800 L; F cylinder: 3600 L.
d. **False** – because the contents are partly in liquid form.
e. **True** – because the gas pressure inside the cylinder is about 54 bar.

2.50 Answers

a. **True** – 'laser': 'light amplification by *stimulated emission* of radiation'.
b. **True** – in population inversion a majority of the entities subject to excitation are in the excited state rather than in the resting state.
c. **False** – remanence is a property of ferromagnetism; see **2.17e**.
d. **False** – gyromagnetic ratio is a feature related to the working of the MRI scanner.
e. **False** – graded-index fibre relates to fibre-optic transmission.

3.1 The following physical phenomena for the scenario

Practice paper 3

3.1 The following are SI units:

   a. Roentgen.
   b. Sievert.
   c. Rad.
   d. Rem.
   e. Gauss.

3.2 The following are derived units under the SI d'Unites:

   a. Pascal.
   b. Radian.
   c. Angstrom.
   d. Tesla.
   e. Curie.

3.3 The following pairs of units denote the same physical quantity:

   a. Mho and siemens.
   b. Joule and calorie.
   c. Becquerel and curie.
   d. Gray and rad.
   e. Sievert and rem.

3.4 The following when relating to the behaviour of light necessarily involve the steradian as a unit of measurement:

   a. Intensity of illumination.
   b. Luminous flux.
   c. Illuminance.
   d. Brightness.
   e. Luminance.

3.5 The following are mere ratios, fractions or percentages and therefore have no units:

   a. Henry's constant.
   b. Avogadro's number.
   c. Dielectric constant.
   d. Atomic number.
   e. Exponential constant.

3.6 The following physical phenomena have the same units as 'force per unit area':

   a. Gravitational constant.
   b. Pressure.
   c. Stress.
   d. Strain.
   e. Surface tension.

3.7 The following units of pressure are independent of changes in gravitational force:

a. Bar.
b. Pascal.
c. Centimetre water.
d. Millimetre mercury.
e. Dynes per square centimetre.

3.8 The following equations in physics are correct:

a. Coulombs × volts = joules.
b. Power × time = energy.
c. Voltage × current = power.
d. Farads × volts = coulombs.
e. Newtons × metres = volts × coulombs.

3.9 The following equations have a quantity A on the left side and a quantity B on the right side such that $A \propto B^4$:

a. Hagen–Poiseuille equation.
b. Nernst equation.
c. Stefan–Boltzmann equation.
d. Van't Hoff equation.
e. Van der Waals equation of state.

3.10 The following relationships are in conformity with the inverse square law:

a. Volume and pressure in respect of Boyle's Law.
b. Flow rate and density in respect of laminar flow of a fluid.
c. Intensity of light and the thickness of its medium of propagation.
d. Latent heat of vaporization of water and the temperature of vaporization.
e. Electrical resistance of a conductor and the temperature of the conductor.

3.11 The following refer to the same thing:

a. Catenation and chelation.
b. Coordination number and valency.
c. Dative covalent bond and coordinate bond.
d. Ionic bond and electrovalent bond.
e. Van der Waals attractions and dipole–dipole attractions.

3.12 The following physical phenomena are, mathematically, exponential in nature:

a. Radioactive decay.
b. Rate of simple diffusion of a gas down a fixed concentration gradient.
c. Variation in the pressure of a fixed mass of gas at constant volume in relation to temperature.
d. The conventional mode of energy discharge from a capacitor.
e. The capacity of an atmosphere to hold water vapour with a rise in temperature.

3.13   The following statements are true:

a. Turbulent flow of fluid in a tube has a parabolic front.
b. The intra-alveolar pressure change during the inspiratory phase of IPPV with a constant flow generator shows a decelerating positive exponential form.
c. The relationship between flow rate and viscosity of a fluid in laminar flow is a rectangular hyperbola.
d. The relationship between temperature and saturation vapour pressure of an inhalational anaesthetic agent is linear.
e. The variation of the volume of a fixed mass of gas at constant pressure is linear with its Celsius temperature.

3.14   The following refer to the same thing:

a. An ideal gas and a perfect gas.
b. An ideal solution and a perfect solution.
c. An ideal liquid and a Newtonian liquid.
d. A noble gas and a rare gas.
e. A non-Newtonian fluid and a thixotropic fluid.

3.15   The osmotic pressure of a solution:

a. Is that pressure of the solution that will cause net outward diffusion of water through its partitioning membrane.
b. Is a colligative property of the solution.
c. Has a direct linear relationship with its osmolarity.
d. Bears a direct linear relationship with the specific gravity (relative density) of the solution.
e. Can be determined by application of the van't Hoff equation.

3.16   The following vary with ambient pressure:

a. Rate of decay of a radioactive isotope.
b. Diamagnetic property of a material.
c. Boiling point of water.
d. Speed of light in a gaseous medium.
e. Saturation vapour pressure of an inhalational anaesthetic agent.

3.17   The Bernoulli phenomenon:

a. Can properly be regarded as an expression of the law of conservation of mechanical energy.
b. Applies only to the flow of gases in tubes.
c. Is a prevailing phenomenon during jet ventilation.
d. Has a significant input into gas flow along anaesthetic rotameter tubes.
e. Can be operational in a co-axial Bain breathing attachment during the inspiratory phase of spontaneous ventilation.

3.18   In the case of turbulent flow of fluids:

a. The flow front has a hyperbolic profile.
b. The density of the fluid is a determinant factor of flow rate.
c. The viscosity of the fluid increases with flow rate.
d. The flow rate is below its 'critical velocity'.
e. The flow rate varies directly with the square of the pressure gradient.

3.19   Adiabatic compression:

a. Is only true for ideal gases.
b. Is also known as the Joule–Kelvin effect.
c. Can occur at the Bodok seal of an anaesthetic machine.
d. Is associated with the functioning of the cryoprobe.
e. Can increase the risk of fire.

3.20   The following gases have a critical temperature above 0 °C:

a. Cyclopropane.
b. Oxygen.
c. Nitrous oxide.
d. Hydrogen.
e. Ozone.

3.21   The following gases can be assayed by the method of mass spectrometry:

a. Oxygen.
b. Argon.
c. Carbon monoxide.
d. Nitrogen dioxide.
e. Ethylene oxide.

3.22   In infrared gas analysis:

a. The method is rapid enough to measure both inspiratory and expiratory gas concentrations.
b. The presence of helium can interfere with carbon dioxide analysis.
c. The presence of water vapour may lead to spurious CO_2 readings.
d. Alcohol, if present, will give spuriously low readings for volatile agents.
e. Changes in atmospheric pressure are likely to alter readings for individual gases.

3.23   Helium can be assayed by the following methods of gas analysis:

a. Mass spectrometry.
b. Raman scattering.
c. Infrared gas analysis.
d. Paramagnetic analysis.
e. Piezo-electric method of gas analysis.

3.24   The presence of the following agents in the patient gas sample has been known to interfere with accurate capnography by the method of infrared analysis:

a. Water vapour.
b. Alcohol vapour.
c. Carbon monoxide.
d. Desflurane.
e. Nitrous oxide.

3.25   In the case of the Clark electrode method of measurement of pO_2:

   a. The two electrodes can be of the same material.
   b. The chemical reaction involving oxygen is analogous to that of the Krebs cycle.
   c. The definitive reaction (that enables determination of the oxygen tension) occurs at the anode.
   d. Electron release is a necessary prerequisite for the assay.
   e. Its performance is unaffected by temperature change.

3.26   The oxygen saturation monitor:

   a. By itself gives an accurate indication of the total oxygen content of blood.
   b. Is an accurate indicator of the adequacy of pulmonary ventilation.
   c. Is an indirect indicator of the fact or otherwise of normocapnia.
   d. Is an immediate true reflection of the adequacy of cardiac output.
   e. Is an indirect index of the partial pressure of oxygen in the arterial blood.

3.27   The following are higher for xenon compared with nitrous oxide:

   a. Molecular weight.
   b. Viscosity.
   c. Boiling point.
   d. MAC.
   e. Critical temperature.

3.28   The following are of the order of a few millivolts:

   a. Amplitude of the waves on a standard ECG.
   b. EMG signals recorded by needle electrodes.
   c. Signals of EEG recordings.
   d. Signals from an ERG (electroretinogram).
   e. Battery voltage of a peripheral nerve stimulator.

3.29   The operational electric energy stimulus of the following equipment has a square wave configuration on graphical display:

   a. An ECT machine.
   b. A peripheral nerve stimulator.
   c. A DC defibrillator.
   d. An isolated diathermy (electrosurgical) machine.
   e. TENS equipment.

3.30   The following function as transducers:

   a. An AC electricity generator.
   b. An electric blanket.
   c. Brown adipose tissue.
   d. A rheostat in an electrical circuit.
   e. A Bair Hugger.

3.31 A better ECG signal (i.e. one that is less attenuated and less interfered with) is obtained if:

a. There is a higher signal-to-noise ratio in the system.
b. The system has a lower amplifier input impedance.
c. The electrode impedance is higher than lower.
d. There is low patient skin impedance.
e. The electrodes are made of different material.

3.32 A higher frequency alternating electric current as opposed to a lower one will:

a. Increase the impedance of a capacitor in the circuit
b. Decrease the reactance of an inductor in the circuit.
c. Increase the impedance of a resistor in the circuit.
d. Decrease the risk of electrocution.
e. Increase the amount of heat energy produced in the system.

3.33 The risk of electrocution from diathermy (electrosurgery) is decreased:

a. If the equipment is of Class I type rather than Class II type.
b. If the frequency of the current is of the order of kilohertz rather than megahertz.
c. If the equipment has incorporated in its circuit an 'isolating capacitor'.
d. If the equipment is 'grounded' rather than 'floating'.
e. If the equipment is 'earthed' rather than not earthed.

3.34 In the case of surgical diathermy (electrocautery):

a. The monopolar mode is the only one that can be used effectively for 'cutting' diathermy.
b. The bipolar mode does not require a diathermy plate.
c. A diathermy plate and its return pathway lead, when in use, are there to earth the patient.
d. The coagulation mode has a higher duty cycle than the cutting mode.
e. The bipolar mode is the one that is conventionally used for TUR prostate surgery.

3.35 Electrical equipment graded as 'Type B':

a. Must necessarily be battery powered.
b. Is 'isolated' from earth.
c. Is safer then 'Type BF' equipment.
d. Is suitable for direct connection to the heart.
e. Has to conform to a more stringent 'allowable patient leakage current' value than 'Type CF' equipment.

3.36   The presence of an inductor in an electrical circuit:

   a. May lead to behaviour of electricity in accordance with Lenz's Law.
   b. Improves the passage of AC electricity in the circuit compared with DC electricity.
   c. Improves the performance of a DC defibrillator.
   d. Interferes with biological electrical signals.
   e. Reduces the likelihood of 'noise'.

3.37   In the case of infrared electromagnetic radiations:

   a. They are invisible.
   b. They are mutagenic.
   c. They are thermogenic.
   d. Glass is generally opaque to them.
   e. They are absorbed by water.

3.38   The following anaesthetic breathing attachments belong to category A in the Mapleson classification:

   a. Magill attachment.
   b. Non-co-axial Bain attachment.
   c. Ayre's T-piece attachment with Jackson Rees modification.
   d. Parallel Lack attachment.
   e. Waters to-and-fro attachment containing a soda lime canister for CO_2 absorption.

3.39   Soda lime used as CO_2 absorbent in a low flow breathing attachment:

   a. Will not function as an absorbent in the absence of sodium hydroxide.
   b. Is more likely to produce carbon monoxide during use if it is dry rather than moist.
   c. Must contain water as an ingredient if it is to function efficiently.
   d. When in use brings about an endothermic chemical reaction.
   e. Produces water as a byproduct of its chemical reactions.

3.40   The Manley MP 3 ventilator:

   a. Is a constant flow generator ventilator.
   b. Is a ventilation rate pre-set ventilator.
   c. Is energized by anaesthetic gases delivered to it at a pressure of 4 bar.
   d. Has an adjustable inspiratory/expiratory time ratio.
   e. Is satisfactory even for patients with poor lung compliance.

3.41   In the case of the Desflurane (Mark 6) vaporizer:

   a. It is a plenum vaporizer.
   b. It is a 'splitting ratio' vaporizer.
   c. It is a 'concentration calibrated' vaporizer.
   d. It works on the 'copper kettle' principle.
   e. Its design can be used effectively to construct vaporizers for other commonly used halogenated inhalational anaesthetic agents.

3.42 **The Waters to-and-fro breathing attachment:**

    a. Is a Mapleson D attachment.

    b. Has a 2 L bag which contains essentially fresh gases when used for spontaneous ventilation with a fresh gas flow comparable with patient minute volume.

    c. Is more efficient than the Bain attachment for spontaneous ventilation.

    d. Can be used satisfactorily with a Nuffield Penlon 200 ventilator for anaesthesia in the artificial ventilation mode.

    e. Suitably modified, can be used effectively for low flow anaesthesia.

3.43 **In the case of oxygen cylinders for medical use:**

    a. They are colour coded with a black body and black and white shoulders.

    b. When full, they have a gauge pressure of 137 bar, no matter the size of the cylinder.

    c. Their G cylinders contain about twice the amount of oxygen as their F cylinders.

    d. They need to have a filling ratio of 0.67 for the UK.

    e. They need to be maintained in the upright position when in use.

3.44 **If a nitrous oxide cylinder is 'bled' at a constant rapid rate:**

    a. The cylinder pressure will diminish proportionately with gas escape, with time.

    b. Frost is likely to form on the outside wall of the cylinder.

    c. The cylinder can stop the exit of the gas if water is a contaminant inside it.

    d. The cylinder contents could suffer from the Poynting effect.

    e. There is a risk of other oxides of nitrogen forming inside the cylinder.

3.45 **In the case of carbon dioxide cylinders on an anaesthetic machine:**

    a. The colour coding of their shoulders is at least partly grey.

    b. They need to have a filling ratio of 0.67 for the UK.

    c. They require a pressure regulator in their gas pathway.

    d. A Bourdon gauge will correctly indicate their contents.

    e. Their pin index positions are 1 and 5.

3.46 **The following are examples of 'dynamic response' in a measuring system:**

    a. Drift.

    b. Hysteresis.

    c. Zero-order response.

    d. First-order response.

    e. Second-order response.

3.47 **The following are phenomena associated with MRI:**

    a. Collimation.

    b. Cavitation.

    c. Remanence.

    d. Precession.

    e. Step-index transmission.

3.48 **A fibre-optic light system:**

a. Operates on the principle of total internal reflection.
b. Needs cladding of another material with a much higher refractive index for it to be functional.
c. Must always have its fibres laid coherently for its proper function.
d. Typically has optical fibres with a diameter of the order of 0.2 mm.
e. Can concentrate fibre light energy to the extent of its being a fire risk.

3.49 **The following are graded according to FCG (French catheter gauge):**

a. Chest drain tubes.
b. Stomach washout tubes.
c. Nasogastric tubes.
d. Urethral catheters.
e. Pulmonary artery flotation catheters.

3.50 **The following statements are true:**

a. The higher the blood–gas partition coefficient of an inhalational anaesthetic agent, the lower the speed of anaesthetic induction.
b. The lower the degree of ionization of an agent, the easier its ability to cross body fluid compartment boundaries.
c. The higher the frequency of alternating electric current, the easier its passage through a capacitor.
d. The lower the frequency of sound waves, the more difficult their passage through a medium.
e. The higher the temperature of a liquid, the lower its latent heat of vaporization.

3.1 Answers

a. False – the roentgen is the former (non-SI) unit of exposure to ionizing radiation. The SI equivalent is coulombs per kilogram. The roentgen is equal to 2.58×10^{-4} C kg^{-1}.

b. True – the unit of 'dose equivalent'. Different types of radiation cause different effects on the body. To make allowance for this the International Commission on Radiological Protection has agreed on a weighted absorbed dose, the *dose equivalent*.

c. False – former non-SI unit of absorbed dose and is equal to 10^{-2} Gray.

d. False – the rem is the pre-SI unit of dose equivalent and is an acronym for *roentgen equivalent man* and is equal to 10^{-2} sievert.

e. False – the gauss is the cgs unit of magnetic flux density. The corresponding SI unit is the tesla. There are 10 000 gauss in a tesla. The earth's magnetic flux density is about 0.6 gauss.

3.2 Answers

a. True – equal to 1 N m^{-2}.

b. False – the radian (like the steradian) is a *supplementary* unit.

c. False – the angstrom is a non-SI unit and is equal to 10^{-10} m or 0.1 nm.

d. True – see **3.1e**.

e. False – the curie is the non-SI unit of the activity of a radionuclide. Its SI equivalent is the becquerel; 1 curie = 3.7×10^{10} Bq.

3.3 Answers

a. True – electrical conductance, the reciprocal of electrical resistance.

b. True – heat. 1 calorie = 4.18 J.

c. True – see **3.2e**.

d. True – see **3.1c**.

e. True – see **3.1d**.

3.4 Answers

a. False – the unit of intensity of illumination is the candela.

b. True – is the rate of flow of luminous energy emitted from a light source (i.e. luminous power) and is measured in lumens, the lumen being that flux which is emitted by a uniform point source of 1 cd in a solid angle of 1 steradian.

c. True – illuminance is the luminous power density incident on a surface. It is expressed in lumens per square metre and therefore involves the steradian in its measurement; see **3.4b**.

d. False – brightness is the subjective evaluation of intensity of illumination, which latter is measured in candela.

e. True – luminance is the luminous intensity per unit area arriving at a surface, leaving the surface or passing through it in a given direction and is expressed in lumens per square metre per steradian.

3.5 Answers

a. **False** – better known as Henry's Law constant, it is the solubility constant of a gas in a liquid and its units are moles (or grams) per unit volume per unit pressure unit (mmHg or kPa).

b. **False** – number of molecules of an element per mole. Note: although referred to as a 'number', Avogadro's number is not a number but a quantity measured per unit mole (mol^{-1}), and therefore more correctly called 'Avogadro's constant'.

c. **True** – same as the relative permittivity of a capacitor.

d. **True** – also known as the proton number, the atomic number is the number of protons in the nucleus of an atom and is denoted by the symbol Z.

e. **True** – it is the exponent of natural logarithms and is equal to 2.718.

3.6 Answers

a. **False** – newtons metre^2 kilogram^{-2}.

b. **True.**

c. **True.**

d. **False** – strain is a ratio and therefore a dimensionless entity.

e. **False** – newtons per metre or joules per square metre.

3.7 Answers

a. **True** – a cgs unit of pressure equal to 10^6 dynes cm^{-2} or 10^5 Pa.

b. **True.**

c. **False.**

d. **False.**

e. **True.**

3.8 Answers

a. **True.**

b. **True** – power (watts) × time (seconds) = energy or work (joules).

c. **True.**

d. **True.**

e. **True** – newtons × metres is 'force × distance', i.e. work; volts × coulombs is joules, which is a unit of work.

3.9 Answers

a. **True** – flow rate ∝ radius^4.

b. **False** – Nernst equation:

E (electrical potential difference across a membrane) $E = \dfrac{RT}{zF} \ln \dfrac{[X]_A}{[X]_B}$.

c. **True** – Stefan–Boltzmann equation: $E = \sigma T^4$, based on the Stefan–Boltzmann Law: the total energy radiated per unit surface area of a black body is proportional to the fourth power of its Kelvin temperature.

d. **False** – van't Hoff equation: $\pi = \rho RT$, where π is the osmotic pressure of a solution, ρ the osmolarity, R the gas constant and T its Kelvin temperature.

e. **False** – van der Waals equation is the variation on the universal gas equation when applied to a non-ideal gas: $(p + \dfrac{a}{V^2})(V - b) = RT$.

3.10 Answers

a. False – the relationship is that of the 'inverse law': $A \propto \frac{1}{B}$; the inverse square law is $A \propto \frac{1}{B^2}$.

b. False – density is not a factor in determining flow rate in respect of laminar flow.

c. True – Beer–Lambert Law.

d. False – although the latent heat of vaporization of water decreases with rising temperature the relationship does not conform to the inverse square law.

e. False – the electrical resistance of a conductor increases with rising temperature.

3.11 Answers

a. False – catenation: simply, the formation of chains of atoms in a compound; chelation: process by which a ligand is coordinated to a metal ion, within an inorganic complex, at two or more points, so that there is a ring of atoms including the metal ions. Chelation occurs in the (i) use of agents to counteract heavy metal poisoning and (ii) use of EDTA to chelate calcium so as to prevent blood clotting.

b. False – valency is the combining power of an atom or radical equal to the number of hydrogen atoms that the atom or radical could combine with. The coordination number is the number of groups, molecules, atoms or ions surrounding a given atom or ion in a compound or crystal. In a square-planar complex the central ion has a coordination number of four. The ferrous iron moiety in the haemoglobin molecule has six coordination sites. Four of them are attached to the nitrogen of a pyrrole group, the fifth to the histidine radical of the α chain and the sixth is the one available for oxygen carriage.

c. True – a dative covalent bond is a covalent bond in which one of the joined atoms supplies both the electrons, as contrasted with a (simple) covalent bond where each atom provides an electron to the bond.

d. True.

e. True – van der Waals forces are weak attractive forces between atoms or molecules and are the forces responsible for the nonideal behaviour of gases and the lattice energy of molecular crystals. Three factors give rise to them: (i) dipole–dipole interactions (i.e. electrostatic attractions) between two molecules with permanent dipole moments; (ii) dipole-induced dipole interactions, where the dipole of one molecule polarizes an adjacent molecule; and (iii) dispersion forces arising from small instantaneous dipoles in atoms.

3.12 Answers

    a. True – a decelerating negative exponential.
    b. False – the change is linear provided the concentration gradient remains unchanged.
    c. False – the change is linear; this is Gay-Lussac's Law.
    d. True.
    e. True – this is in effect the relationship between saturation vapour pressure and temperature. The change is an accelerating growth exponential.

3.13 Answers

    a. False – it is a truncated near-linear front. A parabolic front is characteristic of laminar flow.
    b. False – it is linear. It is a constant pressure generator ventilator that shows a decelerating growth exponential.
    c. True – because the relationship is inverse: $\dot{Q} \propto \dfrac{1}{\eta}$. Wherever a relationship is arithmetically inverse, e.g. in the case of pressure and volume according to Boyle's Law, its graphical representation is a rectangular hyperbola.
    d. False – see **3.12e**.
    e. True – this is Charles' Law.

3.14 Answers

    a. True.
    b. False – an ideal solution obeys Raoult's Law but generally only for dilute solutions. But some solutions obey the Law over a wider range of concentrations and these are called perfect solutions. Therefore, while a perfect solution is also an ideal solution, an ideal solution is not necessarily a perfect solution.
    c. False – an ideal liquid is one that is incompressible. It has no internal frictional forces acting in it, i.e. it is aviscous. A Newtonian fluid is one whose flow is laminar, i.e. it conforms to the Hagen–Poiseuille equation.
    d. True.
    e. False – in a Newtonian fluid the velocity gradient is directly proportional to the shear stress, i.e. $F/A \propto v/d$. Therefore $F/A = \eta\, v/d$, η being viscosity. In the case of a non-Newtonian fluid its velocity gradient is *not* proportional to the shear stress. This means that it has a viscosity that varies with its velocity gradient. Some non-Newtonian liquids have a viscosity that increases as the velocity gradient increases; they are *dilatant* fluids. In others the viscosity increases when the velocity gradient decreases. They are *thixotropic* fluids. In other words, a thixotropic fluid is only one type of non-Newtonian fluid. Blood is a thixotropic fluid. θιξις (thixis): Gk.'touching'.

3.15 Answers

a. False – it is that pressure that would cause a net *inward* diffusion of water, i.e. water is drawn into the compartment with the higher osmotic pressure.

b. True – a *colligative* property is one that is dependent merely on the number of particles of the substance in the solution and not on their mass, charge, valency or reactivity. Colligative properties include osmolarity, vapour pressure, elevation of boiling point and depression of freezing point.

c. True.

d. False – because specific gravity is not a colligative property.

e. True – van't Hoff equation: $\pi = \rho RT$; where π is the osmotic pressure, ρ the density of the fluid, R the universal gas constant, and T the Kelvin temperature. Note the similarity between the van't Hoff equation and the Universal Gas equation, $PV = nRT$.

Therefore $P = \frac{n}{V} RT$; $\frac{n}{V}$ is density, ρ.

3.16 Answers

a. False.

b. False.

c. True.

d. True.

e. False – SVP depends on ambient temperature, but is independent of ambient pressure.

3.17 Answers

a. True.

b. False – applies to 'fluids', i.e. gases and liquids.

c. True.

d. False.

e. True – at the point at which the inner co-axial afferent tube opens into the outer co-axial efferent tube (at the patient end). As the fresh gases leave the inner afferent co-axial tube and enter the outer efferent co-axial tube the Bernoulli phenomenon operates, leading to a slight Venturi effect, aiding the 'downstream' movement of gases in the outer co-axial tube.

3.18 Answers

a. False – a 'truncated' or flat front.

b. True – the flow rate is inversely related to density.

c. False – viscosity plays no part.

d. False – it is above its critical velocity.

e. False – flow rate varies directly with the *square root* of the pressure gradient: $\dot{Q} \propto \sqrt{P}$. Or the pressure gradient is proportional to the square of the flow rate: $P \propto \dot{Q}^2$.

3.19 Answers

a. **False.**
b. **False** – it is adiabatic *decompression* that is known as the Joule–Kelvin effect, also known as the Joule–Thomson effect because Sir William Thomson was ennobled as Lord Kelvin.
c. **True.**
d. **False** – it is adiabatic decompression.
e. **True.**

3.20 Answers

a. **True** – 125 °C.
b. **False** – −118 °C.
c. **True** – 36.4 °C.
d. **False** – −239 °C.
e. **False** – −12 °C.

3.21 Answers

a. **True.**
b. **True.**
c. **True.**
d. **True.**
e. **True.**

Note: all gases can be assayed by mass spectrometry.

3.22 Answers

a. **True.**
b. **True** – it has been found that the presence of helium 79% in oxygen leads to under-reading of CO_2.
c. **True** – because water vapour absorbs infrared radiations.
d. **False** – spuriously high readings.
e. **True** – because the reading is of 'partial pressures', any change in atmospheric pressure will affect the value.

3.23 Answers

a. **True.**
b. **False.**
c. **False.**
d. **True** – helium is paramagnetic, but only very slightly compared with oxygen.
e. **False.**

3.24 Answers

a. **True.**
b. **True.**
c. **True** – because the majority of absorption of infrared for carbon monoxide is at 4.7 μm (that for CO_2 is 4.3 μm)
d. **True** – desflurane has been known to interfere with accurate CO_2 estimation by infrared analysis, but the effect is insignificant.
e. **True** – absorption band for N_2O is 4.5 μm. However, this is electronically corrected for in conventional infrared analysis.

3.25 Answers

a. False.
b. True.
c. False – it occurs at the cathode; it is: $O_2 + 2H_2O + 4e = 4OH^-$.
d. True – see **c** above.
e. False.

3.26 Answers

a. False – the haemoglobin content also needs to be known.
b. False.
c. False.
d. False.
e. True.

3.27 Answers

a. True – xenon: 131; nitrous oxide: 44.
b. True – xenon: (at 20 °C) 0.0227 mPa s; nitrous oxide (at 20 °C) 0.0147 mPa s.
c. False – xenon: −108 °C; nitrous oxide: −88.6 °C.
d. False – xenon: 71; nitrous oxide: 105.
e. False – xenon: 16.5 °C; nitrous oxide: 36.4 °C.

3.28 Answers

a. True.
b. True.
c. False – microvolts.
d. False – about 0.5 mV.
e. False.

3.29 Answers

a. True.
b. True.
c. False – traditionally it was a damped sine wave, but may be monophasic or biphasic and also saw-toothed, truncated or rectilinear.
d. False – it is a sine wave.
e. True.

3.30 Answers

a. True – converts chemical energy (oil or petroleum) into electrical energy.
b. True – converts electrical energy into heat energy.
c. True – converts chemical energy into thermal energy.
d. False – merely adjusts the impedance and therefore the current in a circuit.
e. True – converts electrical energy into thermal energy.

3.31 Answers

a. **True.**
b. **False.**
c. **False.**
d. **True.**
e. **False.**

3.32 Answers

a. **False** – will decrease the impedance.
b. **False** – will increase the reactance.
c. **False** – it will not affect the impedance of a resistor.
d. **True.**
e. **False.**

3.33 Answers

a. **False.**
b. **False** – a megahertz frequency electric current will provide greater protection from electrocution than a kilohertz frequency current.
c. **True.**
d. **False.**
e. **True.**

3.34 Answers

a. **True.**
b. **True.**
c. **False.**
d. **False** – duty cycle: coagulation mode: c. 5–20%; cutting mode: 95–100%. *Duty cycle*: the ratio, expressed as a percentage, of the time for which a unit is activated to the total duration of the on–off cycle of a periodically repeated operation.
e. **False** – monopolar mode.

3.35 Answers

a. **False** – may be mains powered or possess an internal power source, i.e. a battery.
b. **False** – it is 'Type BF' equipment that is isolated from earth.
c. **False** – 'Type BF' is safer for reason stated in **b** above.
d. **False** – equipment suitable for direct connection to the heart must be of 'Type CF'.
e. **False** – for reason stated in **d** above.

3.36 Answers

a. **True** – the inductor induces a 'back EMF' in the circuit which opposes the primary EMF.
b. **False.**
c. **True** – by 'levelling out' the current energy delivery through the heart.
d. **False.**
e. **False.**

Note: Lenz's Law (after Heinrich Lenz [1804–1865]): An induced electric current always flows in a direction such that it opposes the change producing it. This is essentially an expression of the Law of Conservation of Energy.

3.37 Answers

a. **True.**
b. **False.**
c. **True.**
d. **True.**
e. **True.**

3.38 Answers

a. **True.**
b. **False** – Bain non-co-axial is a Mapleson D.
c. **False.**
d. **True.**
e. **False.**

3.39 Answers

a. **False** – it will function, but at a much slower rate of reaction. The NaOH acts as a catalyst.
b. **True.**
c. **True** – water is essential for the first reaction:
$CO_2 + H_2O \rightarrow H_2CO_3$.
d. **False** – an exothermic reaction.
e. **True.**

3.40 Answers

a. **False** – constant pressure generator ventilator.
b. **False** – it is the tidal volume that is pre-set. The rate is equal to the fresh gas flow rate divided by the tidal volume.
c. **False** – its driving energy is provided by the fresh gas flow, which is delivered at a pressure of about one-third bar.
d. **True.**
e. **False** – patients with poor lung compliance need a flow generator ventilator.

3.41 Answers

a. True.
b. False – it is a 'copper kettle' type vaporizer.
c. False – a 'concentration calibrated' vaporizer is the same as a 'splitting ratio' type vaporizer.
d. True.
e. True.

3.42 Answers

a. False – Mapleson B or C, depending on whether it contains a length of corrugated hose between the APL valve and breathing bag, in which case it is a C.
b. False – a mixture of fresh and exhaled gases.
c. True.
d. False.
e. True – by incorporating a soda lime canister between the patient and breathing bag. It has been used as such in the past.

3.43 Answers

a. False – black body and white shoulders.
b. True.
c. False – F cylinder: 1360 L; G cylinder: 3400 L.
d. False – oxygen cylinders are not required to conform to the 'filling ratio' requirement because their contents are entirely gaseous even under pressure.
e. False.

3.44 Answers

a. False – because, as gas escapes, liquid will vaporize to make up the shortfall, and the pressure will thus be restored. But the pressure will progressively diminish, albeit only slightly, because of the drop in temperature of the contents, in accordance with Gay-Lussac's Law.
b. True – because of the temperature fall.
c. True – because the fall in temperature can be low enough to cause freezing of any contaminant water, which will then block the exit port of the cylinder.
d. False.
e. False.

3.45 Answers

a. True – both shoulders and body are grey.
b. True.
c. True – because the cylinder contents are at c. 50 bar, which has to be reduced to 4 bar before the gas reaches the CO_2 flowmeter.
d. False.
e. False – the positions are 1 and 6.

3.46 Answers

a. **True.**
b. **True.**
c. **False.**
d. **False.**
e. **False.**

3.47 Answers

a. **False** – collimation (i.e. nondivergence of light beam) is a feature of laser light.
b. **False** – cavitation is a phenomenon associated with ultrasound waves.
c. **True** – remanence is the presence of some residual magnetic flux in a ferromagnet even after the magnetizing force has been removed.
d. **True** – precession is the 'wobbling' of the hydrogen protons under the influence of the radiofrequency EMR wave stimulus.
e. **False** – step-index transmission is a feature of fibre-optic transmission.

3.48 Answers

a. **True.**
b. **False** – the cladding must have a lower refractive index.
c. **False** – coherence in fibre layout is only necessary if the light is to transmit a picture, but not necessary if the light is merely for illumination.
d. **False** – diameter c. 20 micrometres.
e. **True.**

3.49 Answers

a. **True.**
b. **True.**
c. **True.**
d. **True.**
e. **True.**

3.50 Answers

a. **True.**
b. **True.**
c. **True.**
d. **False** – it is easier.
e. **True.**

Practice paper 4

4.1 The following are derived units under the SI Units system:

    a. Newton.
    b. Ampere.
    c. Steradian.
    d. Electron-volt.
    e. Stokes.

4.2. The radian is:

    a. A fundamental unit under the SI nomenclature.
    b. A dimensionless entity.
    c. The SI unit of solid angle.
    d. The unit of measurement of angular displacement.
    e. The mode of measurement of displacement in simple harmonic motion.

4.3 The following statements are true:

    a. *Ampere* is the unit of quantity of electricity flowing in a circuit.
    b. *Lumen* is the unit of intensity of illumination.
    c. Surface tension may correctly be expressed as joules per square metre.
    d. *Poise* is the SI unit of kinematic viscosity.
    e. *Tesla* is the unit of magnetic flux.

4.4 The following are units of measurement of energy:

    a. Joule.
    b. Calorie.
    c. Electron-volt.
    d. Erg.
    e. Coulomb.

4.5 The following refer to the same thing:

    a. Fundamental quantity and base quantity.
    b. Supplementary units and derived units.
    c. Thermodynamic temperature and Kelvin temperature.
    d. Electrical impedance and electrical resistance.
    e. Resistance and elastance (in relation to gases in the respiratory system).

4.6 The following refer to the same thing:

    a. Tonicity and osmolarity in relation to body compartment fluids.
    b. Thermodynamic temperature scale and absolute temperature scale.
    c. Critical temperature and Boyle temperature.
    d. London forces and van der Waals forces.
    e. Natural logarithms and Napierian logarithms.

4.7 The following are 'dimensionless entities' i.e. they are mere ratios, fractions or percentages:

a. Substitution index.
b. Therapeutic index.
c. Refractive index.
d. Cardiac index.
e. Quetelet index.

4.8 The following are approximately equal to a pressure of one newton per square metre:

a. Pascal.
b. Dyne per square centimetre.
c. Torr.
d. Millibar.
e. One centimetre water pressure

4.9 The following have the same physical units as does quantum of energy:

a. Pressure × volume.
b. Voltage × coulombs.
c. Watts × seconds.
d. Force × area.
e. Electrical capacitance × electrical resistance.

4.10 The following relationships are linear in nature:

a. Variation of volume with temperature of a fixed mass of gas at constant pressure.
b. Change of intensity of sound with distance of propagation of the sound wave.
c. Relationship between haematocrit and blood viscosity.
d. Variation of flow rate in turbulent flow with pressure gradient.
e. Frequency of AC electricity and the threshold current required to induce ventricular fibrillation.

4.11 The following when graphically depicted take the form of a rectangular hyperbola:

a. Variation of pressure and volume of a fixed mass of gas in accordance with Boyle's Law.
b. Relationship between saturation vapour pressure of an inhalational anaesthetic agent and temperature.
c. Strength–duration curve of a stimulus of electrical depolarization of a cell membrane.
d. Relationship between the specific density of 'physiological' urine and its osmolarity.
e. Variation of electrical conductance of a semiconductor with its temperature.

4.12 **The following have an osmolarity of approximately 1 mosmol ml^{-1} of solution:**

a. 1 mole of glucose dissolved in 1 L of solution.
b. 60 g of urea dissolved in one litre of water.
c. A molar solution of sodium chloride.
d. An 8.4% solution of sodium bicarbonate.
e. 1 g of potassium chloride dissolved in 500 ml of solution.

4.13 **In the case of electromagnetic radiations (EMRs):**

a. They all travel at the speed of light.
b. They can exist only at temperatures above 0 kelvin.
c. They have a plane of propagation at right angles to that of their amplitude.
d. They are more likely to be mutagenic the longer their wavelengths.
e. They possess energy levels in direct linear proportion to their Celsius temperature.

4.14 **The operational frequencies of the following are of the order of megahertz or higher:**

a. Diathermy (electrosurgical) unit.
b. US scanner.
c. 'Harmonic scalpel' (ultrasound when used for achieving surgical haemostasis).
d. Micro-wave oven.
e. Larmor frequency of MRI scanner.

4.15 **The following are graded according to SWG (steel wire gauge):**

a. Hypodermic needle.
b. Quadruple central venous catheter.
c. Whitacre spinal needle.
d. Tracheal suction catheter.
e. Intra-arterial cannulae.

4.16 **The following features are common to the Clark Cell and the Fuel Cell as devices used for oxygen analysis:**

a. They both have a platinum cathode.
b. They both require an 'external' potential difference.
c. They both measure oxygen tension.
d. They are both temperature sensitive.
e. Both methods of analysis can be affected by the presence of inhalational agents.

4.17 **In the process of loss of body heat by radiation:**

a. It usually accounts for less than 25% of total body heat loss.
b. It is predominantly in the form of ultraviolet radiations.
c. It can occur even if the human body is placed in a vacuum.
d. It can occur against a temperature gradient.
e. Other things being equal, the loss is greater in a dark skinned person than in a fair skinned person.

4.18 **The following increase with a rise in temperature:**

a. Solubility of a gas in a liquid.
b. Saturation vapour pressure of an inhalational anaesthetic agent.
c. Viscosity of a liquid.
d. Diamagnetic property of a material.
e. Rate of decay of a radioactive isotope.

4.19 **The normal duration of discharge of the current stimulus from the following devices is under 1 ms:**

a. Peripheral nerve stimulator.
b. Cardiac pacemaker.
c. DC defibrillator when operational in 'manual' mode.
d. TENS machine for pain relief.
e. Current discharge during electroconvulsive therapy.

4.20 **The following statements are true with respect to electricity:**

a. Reactance is present in circuits containing capacitors and inductors, but not resistors.
b. Resistance is a component of impedance in relation to an AC circuit.
c. The presence of a capacitor in an AC circuit results in a phase difference between voltage and current.
d. A perfect capacitor in an AC circuit has resistance but no reactance.
e. A perfect inductor in an AC circuit has reactance but no resistance.

4.21 **DC electricity, as opposed to AC electricity, is the preferred mode for the following:**

a. Current energy for synchronized cardioconversion.
b. Electrical stimulus for the peripheral nerve stimulator.
c. Coagulation mode for diathermy (electrosurgery) during surgery of TUR prostate.
d. Heat treatment as part of physiotherapy.
e. Use of a SELV machine for electrocautery.

4.22 **Other things being equal, protection from electrocution from operating theatre equipment is enhanced if the equipment is:**

a. SELV energized than otherwise.
b. Provided with an 'isolation transformer'.
c. Type B rather than type BF.
d. Is earthed rather than isolated.
e. Is 'defibrillator protected' rather than not so protected.

4.23 **The following are attributes associated with the activity of diathermy (electrosurgery):**

a. Duty cycle.
b. Blending.
c. Collimation.
d. Return electrode monitoring.
e. Coercivity.

4.24 The following are examples of transducers:

a. The human retina.
b. A step-up transformer.
c. The heating element of an electric kettle.
d. The *phosphor* in a fluorescent ('strip') light tube.
e. A sound microphone.

4.25 The following are by definition transducers:

a. A dry cell battery.
b. Brown adipose tissue.
c. A microwave oven.
d. A mutual induction solenoid.
e. The inductor in a DC defibrillator circuit.

4.26 The following are associated with the behaviour of EMRs (electromagnetic radiations):

a. Peltier effect.
b. Larmor frequency.
c. Wien constant.
d. van't Hoff factor.
e. Avogadro's number.

4.27 The energy waves employed in the following modes of imaging are recognized as capable of inducing mutagenesis in human cells:

a. Infrared imaging.
b. Conventional radiography.
c. Computerized axial tomography.
d. Ultrasonography.
e. Nuclear magnetic resonance imaging.

4.28 In the case of ultra violet EM radiations:

a. They are generally invisible.
b. They are mutagenic.
c. They can be absorbed by oxygen.
d. They are absorbed by glass.
e. They are absorbed by ozone.

4.29 Helium has an essential role in the following for the reasons stated against each:

a. As a supercoolant in the MRI scanner because it is the only gas that still remains liquid at near 0 kelvin.
b. Management of lower airway obstruction because of the low density of the agent.
c. Functioning of the carbon dioxide laser because the agent helps maintain 'population inversion'.
d. As an anaesthetic carrier gas during laser surgery on the throat because of its inertness.
e. As a substitute for nitrogen in breathing gas mixtures in deep sea diving apparatus so as to prevent the 'bends'.

4.30 Oxygen for medical use:

a. Is now manufactured by the Brin process.
b. Can be stored as a liquid before supply for clinical use.
c. When stored in a cylinders manifold is usually in size H cylinders.
d. Is more than 99% pure when provided for medical use.
e. Has a critical temperature of about 154 kelvin.

4.31 Oxygen can be measured by the following methods of gas analysis:

a. Mass spectrometry.
b. Raman scattering.
c. Infrared gas analysis.
d. Paramagnetic analysis.
e. Piezo-electric method of gas analysis.

4.32 Nitrous oxide:

a. Is obtained from natural gas for medical purposes.
b. Has a higher critical temperature than carbon dioxide.
c. In aqueous solution alters the pH of water.
d. Even when under pressure has been available in gaseous form at room temperature when in mixture with other gases.
e. Is prone to decompose into nitrogen dioxide with time during storage in cylinders.

4.33 A Newtonian fluid:

a. By definition is one that is incompressible.
b. Has no internal frictional forces acting in it.
c. Is one in which the viscosity is independent of its shear rate.
d. Is one in which the shear rate is directly proportional to its shear stress.
e. In its behaviour conforms to the Hagen–Poiseuille Law.

4.34 The following thermometers measure temperature by detecting a change in the coefficient of expansion of a material:

a. Mercury clinical thermometer.
b. Gas thermometer.
c. Alcohol thermometer.
d. Thermometer based on a 'bimetallic strip'.
e. Bourdon gauge type of thermometer.

4.35 The following describe the behaviour of gases when dissolving in liquids:

a. Graham's Law
b. Henry's Law.
c. Bunsen coefficient.
d. Fick principle.
e. Bernoulli phenomenon.

4.36 **The following items of equipment operate by means of flap valves rather than spring-loaded valves:**

a. The afferent and efferent limbs of an anaesthetic low flow circle breathing attachment.
b. The 'spill over' valve in the vicinity of the breathing bag attachment on an anaesthetic circle breathing circuit.
c. Ambu valve.
d. Ruben valve.
e. The adjustable pressure limiting valve of a Magill (Mapleson A) anaesthetic breathing attachment.

4.37 **The following devices measure gas flow by utilizing the variable orifice principle:**

a. Anaesthetic machine CO_2 flowmeter tube.
b. Wall point O_2 flowmeter tube.
c. Wright respirometer.
d. Wright peak flowmeter.
e. Pitot tube.

4.38 **The following anaesthetic breathing attachments can be conveniently converted for low flow anaesthesia by incorporation of a soda lime canister for CO_2 absorption:**

a. Magill attachment.
b. Lack co-axial attachment.
c. Parallel Lack attachment.
d. Bain co-axial attachment.
e. Waters to-and-fro breathing attachment.

4.39 **Adiabatic expansion:**

a. Is a phenomenon limited to non-ideal gases.
b. Is associated with the industrial production of oxygen for medical use.
c. Requires the overcoming of van der Waals forces.
d. Can occur at the Bodok seal of an anaesthetic machine.
e. Is usually accompanied by an increase in thermal energy.

4.40 **The following are relevant to magnetic resonance imaging:**

a. Thermal jostling.
b. Population inversion.
c. Time–gain compensation.
d. Gyromagnetic ratio.
e. Free induction decay.

4.41 **Surface tension:**

a. Is the energy required per unit area to maintain the integrity of a liquid surface.
b. Is usually expressed in newtons per square metre.
c. Has a high value for water because of the presence of London forces.
d. Is measured by means of a viscometer.
e. Is reduced in the lung because of the presence of di-palmitoyl choline.

4.42 **Water vapour in an anaesthetic low flow circle breathing attachment which provides for CO_2 absorption by soda lime:**

    a. Can be part of the water inherent in soda lime.
    b. Is essential for the reaction of CO_2 with soda lime.
    c. Is a by-product of the chemical reaction involving CO_2 absorption by soda lime.
    d. Usually accumulates in the soda lime from the patient's exhalations.
    e. Can increase the likelihood of carbon monoxide formation.

4.43 **The gas flowmeter tubes on anaesthetic machines:**

    a. Can properly be referred to as constant pressure differential, variable orifice flow gauges.
    b. Have increasingly widening bores from top to bottom.
    c. May safely be interchanged between the different gases.
    d. Need not be rendered antistatic, now that no explosive inhalational anaesthetic agents are in use.
    e. Are more likely to have sticking bobbins at high gas flow rates than at low gas flow rates.

4.44 **The Bodok seal on an anaesthetic machine:**

    a. Is situated downstream of the pressure regulator valve:
    b. Must necessarily be made of non-combustible material.
    c. Usually has a neoprene component as part of its structure.
    d. Must be capable of withstanding the effects of adiabatic expansion of gases.
    e. Is not essential if the machine were provided solely with piped gases at 4 bar pressures.

4.45 **A size J oxygen cylinder:**

    a. When full has a gauge pressure the same as a size D oxygen cylinder.
    b. Has an empty weight approximately twice that of an empty size G cylinder.
    c. When full contains four times as much oxygen as a size E cylinder.
    d. Normally has a pin index outlet.
    e. Is the one that is normally provided for ward use.

4.46 **In the case of entonox cylinders:**

    a. Their colour coding includes shoulders that are at least partly blue.
    b. Their largest size in the UK is J.
    c. They are available with pin index heads right through the range of cylinder size.
    d. Their contents can be determined only by weighing the cylinder.
    e. Their F size cylinders contain four times as much of the gases as their D size cylinders.

4.47 The following phenomena can occur in a vacuum:

a. Transmission of light.
b. Passage of sound waves.
c. Disintegration of a radionuclide.
d. Existence of a magnetic field.
e. Transfer of heat.

4.48 The following are non-linear:

a. Graduations on an anaesthetic flowmeter tube.
b. Markings on a mercury sphygmomanometer.
c. Divisions on a Bourdon pressure gauge on an anaesthetic machine.
d. Markings on an airway pressure gauge on the efferent limb of a circle breathing attachment.
e. The % markings on a Mark 4 sevoflurane anaesthetic vaporizer.

4.49 A rise in temperature will lead to the following:

a. Increase in electrical resistance of a semiconductor.
b. Decrease in electrical resistance of an insulator.
c. Increase in the ferromagnetism of a ferromagnetic body.
d. Decrease in the solubility of a gas in a liquid.
e. Increase in the radioactive decay of a radionuclide.

4.50 The following statements are true:

a. A racemic mixture is optically inactive.
b. *Cis–trans* isomerism necessarily requires the presence of a carbon–carbon double bond in the configuration of the isomer.
c. *R*-configuration agents are necessarily dextro-rotatory.
d. Diastereomers are stereo-isomers which are not mirror images of one another.
e. Enantiomers differ from one another only with respect to chirality.

4.1 Answers

a. True.
b. False – ampere is the *base* unit of electric current.
c. False – the steradian (like the radian) is a *supplementary* unit.
d. False – the electron-volt (eV) is a non-SI unit of energy.
e. False – the stokes is the non-SI unit of kinematic viscosity.

4.2 Answers

a. False – it is a *supplementary* unit; see **4.1c**.
b. True – because it is not expressible in the units of mass (M), length (L) and time (T), the three fundamental units. But since it is a 'unit' that measures a *quantity* (plane angle) it should be regarded as having 'dimensions'. But, nevertheless, the radian and the steradian are regarded as dimensionless entities.
c. False – it is the SI unit of plane angle, the steradian being the SI unit of solid angle.
d. True.
e. True.

4.3 Answers

a. False – the ampere is a 'rating', i.e. the rate of passage of electrical energy (coulombs) in a circuit. Therefore coulombs/seconds = amperes.
b. False – the lumen is the unit of rate of flow of luminous energy from a light source. The unit of intensity of illumination is the candela.
c. True – surface tension is conventionally expressed in newtons per metre, which is the same as joules per square metre.
d. False – poise is not an SI unit and in any case it is the (non-SI) unit of dynamic viscosity. The stokes is the (non-SI) unit of kinematic viscosity. Kinematic viscosity is dynamic viscosity divided by density: $\frac{\eta}{\rho}$.
e. False – tesla is the unit of magnetic flux density. The unit of magnetic flux is the weber. Therefore, tesla = weber metre^{-2}.

4.4 Answers

a. True – the SI unit of energy. It is the work done when a force of 1 N acts through a distance of 1 m.
b. True – a non-SI unit of energy. It is the amount of heat energy required to raise the temperature of 1 g of water by 1 °C; 1 calorie = 4.18 J.
c. True – a non-SI unit. The energy required to move an electron through a potential difference of 1 V. It is equal to 1.602×10^{-19} J.
d. True – the erg is the cgs unit of energy, i.e. the work done when a force of 1 dyne acts through a distance of 1 cm. 1 J = 10^7 ergs.
e. False – the coulomb is the unit of electrical charge.

4.5 Answers

a. **False** – there are three *fundamental quantities*: mass, length and time. The three fundamental quantities as well as current, temperature, amount of substance and intensity of illumination are the seven base quantities.

b. **False** – see **4.1c**.

c. **True.**

d. **False** – impedance is a generic term for the opposition to flow of electric current in a circuit and includes resistance and reactance.

e. **False** – the units of resistance, which is the reciprocal of conductance, are cmH_2O pressure per millilitre per second; the units of elastance, which is the reciprocal of compliance, are centimetres of water pressure per millilitre.

4.6 Answers

a. **False** – osmolarity measures the concentration of all the (solute) particles in a solution. Tonicity is a measure of only those particles capable of exerting an osmotic force across the cell membrane. In other words tonicity is *effective* osmolarity and is that part of the total osmolarity that is due to the *effective* osmoles.

b. **True.**

c. **False** – critical temperature: the temperature above which a gas cannot be liquefied by pressure alone. Boyle temperature: the temperature at which a gas most closely approximates to an ideal gas.

d. **False** – London forces are just one type of van der Waals force. They are present in all molecules and are weak attractive forces resulting from temporary dipoles that result from erratic motions of electrons even in molecules that have no permanent polarity.

e. **True** – named after the Scottish mathematician John Napier (1550–1616).

4.7 Answers

a. **True** – also known as the degree of substitution, the substitution index is the ratio of hydroxyl moieties in glucose units substituted with hydroxyethyl groups to the total number of glucose molecules. The substitution index is a measure of the resistance to in vivo hydrolysis of hydroxyethyl starches. The higher the substitution index of hydroxyethyl starches, the longer their plasma volume expanding capacity.

b. **True** – ratio between the maximum tolerated dose and the minimum curative dose.

c. **True** – the ratio of the speed of light in one medium to that in an adjacent medium. It is of importance in fibre-optic transmission of light.

d. **False** – cardiac output in litres per minute per square metre of body surface area.

e. **False** – the Quetelet index is the same as the body mass index and therefore has the units kilograms per $metre^2$. It is named after Lambert Adolphe Jacques Quetelet (1796–1874), the Belgian astronomer and statistician.

4.8 Answers

a. True – it is exactly equal because the definition of the pascal is 1 N m^{-2} of area.
b. False – 1 dyne cm^{-2} is equivalent to 0.1 N m^{-2}.
c. False – 1 torr = 1 mmHg, which is 133 Pa (newtons per square metre).
d. False – 1000 millibars = 1 atmosphere = $100\,000$ Pa. Therefore 1 millibar = 100 Pa, i.e 100 N m^{-2}.
e. False – 1 atmosphere = 1000 cmH$_2$O = $100\,000$ Pa. Therefore, 1 cmH$_2$O = 100 Pa, i.e. 100 N m^{-2}.

4.9 Answers

a. True – pressure (in pascals) $\times$ volume (in metres^3) = joules.
b. True – volts $\times$ coulombs = joules.
c. True.
d. False – it is force $\times$ distance that is equal to work; newtons $\times$ metres = joules.
e. False – capacitance (farads) $\times$ resistance (ohms) = time (seconds).

4.10 Answers

a. True – this is Charles' Law.
b. False – the relationship obeys the inverse square law and is therefore exponential in nature.
c. False – the relationship is one of an accelerating growth exponential.
d. False – $\dot{Q} \propto \sqrt{P}$. Therefore the relationship is exponential.
e. False – the relationship is a near hyperbola.

4.11 Answers

a. True.
b. False – it is an accelerating growth exponential.
c. True.
d. False – it is linear, but if the urine were 'unphysiological', i.e. it contained excess protein, the relationship would be exponential, because the increase in specific density would be out of proportion to the increase in osmolarity.
e. False – it is an accelerating growth exponential.

Note: whenever there is a simple inverse relationship between variables, i.e. $A \propto \dfrac{1}{B}$, its graphical representation takes the form of a rectangular hyperbola.

4.12 Answers

a. True – 1 mol of glucose in 1 L of solution is the same as 1 mmol ml^{-1}. Since glucose is an undissociated molecule it will have an osmolarity of 1 mosmol ml^{-1}.

b. True – 60 g of urea is 1 mol because its molecular weight is 60. Like, glucose (see **a** above) this is equal to 1 mmol ml^{-1}, and since urea is an undissociated molecule, the osmolarity is 1 mosmol ml^{-1}.

c. False – a molar solution contains 1 g mol in 1 L of solution, i.e. 1 mmol ml^{-1} of solution. However, sodium chloride dissociates. Therefore the osmolarity will be greater than 1 mosmol ml^{-1}.

d. False – 8.4% sodium bicarbonate has 84 mg of the agent per millilitre of solution. This is equal to 1 mmol ml^{-1} because the molecular weight of sodium bicarbonate is 84. However, like sodium chloride, sodium bicarbonate is dissociated. Therefore its osmolarity is more than 1 mosmol ml^{-1}.

e. False – the molecular weight of potassium chloride is 75 (atomic weight of potassium is 39 and that of chlorine is c. 36. One gram of KCl in 500 ml is 2 g in 1 L; 2 g of KCl is $\frac{2000}{75}$, i.e. 26.7 mmol. Therefore the osmolarity of KCl (were it to be undissociated) would be $\frac{1000}{26.7}$, i.e. 0.037 mosmol L^{-1}. If the KCl were fully dissociated the osmolarity would be 0.074 mosmol ml^{-1}.

4.13 Answers

a. True – 299 792 458 m s^{-1} in a vacuum.

b. True.

c. True – cf. sound waves whose plane of propagation is the same as that of their amplitude.

d. False – they are more likely to be mutagenic the shorter their wavelengths.

e. False – their energy levels are proportional to the fourth power of their Kelvin temperatures.

4.14 Answers

a. True – 3–3.5 MHz.

b. True – c. 1–3.5 MHz.

c. False – the frequency is about 50 kHz.

d. True – c. 2.54 GHz.

e. True – Larmor frequency: the frequency of precession of hydrogen protons during MRI scanning. They are normally in the radiofrequency range.

4.15 Answers

a. True.
b. False – FCG.
c. True.
d. False – FCG.
e. True.

Note: there are two gauges encountered in relation to medical devices. SWG (steel wire gauge) is an 'arbitrary' number and a dimensionless entity. It is based on the number of 'steel wires' of the same diameter as the device in question that can be accommodated in a standard hollow cylinder. This means that the higher the number, the narrower the device. SWG normally applies to needles, cannulae and epidural catheters and is 'dimensionless', i.e. it has no units. The other gauge is FCG (French catheter gauge). This is the external circumference of the device in millimetres. Therefore it is unitized. It normally applies to tracheostomy tubes, suction catheters, stomach tubes, chest drains, etc. It also now applies to quadruple lumen venous catheters. The 'odd one out' is tracheal tubes which are graded according to their internal diameter.

4.16 Answers

a. False – Clark cell: silver/silver chloride anode, platinum cathode; fuel cell: lead anode, gold cathode.
b. False – Clark cell requires an external potential difference source, the fuel cell does not.
c. True.
d. True.
e. True – the Clark cell is affected by the presence of halothane, the fuel cell by nitrous oxide.

4.17 Answers

a. False – accounts for 40–50% of body heat loss.
b. False – in the form of infrared radiations.
c. True – radiation is the only mode of heat transfer that can occur in a vacuum.
d. False – evaporation is the only means by which heat can be lost against a temperature gradient.
e. False – when it comes to loss of body heat all human beings, irrespective of skin colour, act as 'black body radiators'.

4.18 Answers

a. False – it decreases.
b. True.
c. False – viscosity of a liquid decreases with temperature rise.
d. False – diamagnetism is not temperature dependent.
e. False – temperature change does not affect the rate of decay of a radionuclide.

4.19 Answers

    a. True – c. 200–300 μs.
    b. False – usually about 2 ms.
    c. False – 3–5 ms.
    d. True – about 50–300 μs.
    e. False – up to 4 ms.

4.20 Answers

    a. True – reactance is the opposition to the flow of electricity in an AC circuit containing capacitors and/or inductors.
    b. True – impedance is a generic term that embraces all types of opposition to current flow in electrical circuits.
    c. True – the current precedes voltage by 90 degrees.
    d. False – it has reactance but no resistance.
    e. True.

4.21 Answers

    a. True.
    b. True.
    c. False.
    d. False.
    e. True.

4.22 Answers

    a. True – SELV means 'safety extra low voltage'.
    b. True.
    c. False – Type B: Class I, II or III electrical equipment, mains powered or energized by an internal power source. The equipment must provide adequate protection against electric shock, especially with reference to allowable leakage currents. Type BF: equipment whose parts that are applied to the patient are isolated from all other parts of the equipment to the extent that allowable leakage current under single fault conditions is not exceeded even when 1.1 times the rated mains voltage is applied between the applied parts and earth. Note: neither Type B nor Type BF equipment is suitable for direct connection to the heart.
    d. False.
    e. False – the purpose of 'defibrillator protection' is to protect any equipment (such as an ECG machine) connected to a patient from damage by the electrical energy of defibrillation. Its role is not to protect the patient or bystanders.

4.23 Answers

a. **True** – duty cycle: the ratio, expressed as a percentage, of the time for which a unit is activated to the total duration of the on–off cycle of a periodically repeated operation.

b. **True** – 'mixing' of cutting and coagulation modes of diathermy so that the two functions can be used by the surgeon simultaneously.

c. **False** – collimation is a property of laser light, i.e. the nondivergence of the light beam.

d. **True** – constant surveillance of the adequacy of contact of the diathermy plate to the patient skin so as to ensure a low 'current density' at the patient–plate interface at all times.

e. **False** – coercivity is a phenomenon associated with ferromagnetism. It is the magnetic field strength required to reduce the residual magnetic flux density in a magnetic material to 0.

4.24 Answers

a. **True** – converts light energy to electrical energy.

b. **False** – merely ups the voltage.

c. **True** – converts electrical energy to heat energy.

d. **False** – the purpose of a *phosphor* is to alter the EMR waves to those within the visible part of the spectrum; so it merely changes the frequency of the EMRs.

e. **True** – converts sound energy into an electrical signal.

4.25 Answers

a. **True** – converts chemical energy into electrical energy.

b. **True** – converts chemical energy into heat energy.

c. **True** – converts electrical energy into heat energy.

d. **False.**

e. **False.**

4.26 Answers

a. **False** – Peltier effect: change in temperature that occurs at the junction of two dissimilar metals in an electrical circuit when an electric current passes through it. If the current is reversed there is a fall in temperature.

b. **True** – Larmor frequency: the frequency of EMRs (in this case in the radiofrequency range) applied to the nucleus of hydrogen atoms in a magnetic field so as to increase the precession of the protons of the atoms. It is a preliminary step in the process of MRI.

c. **True** – Wien's Displacement Law states that the wavelength of peak emission of EMRs is inversely proportional to their absolute temperature; therefore, $\lambda \propto \frac{1}{T}$; therefore, $\lambda = w \times \frac{1}{T}$, where λ is the wavelength in metres, T the temperature in Kelvin, and w the Wien constant, which has the value 2.9×10^{-3} m K.

d. **False** – van't Hoff factor: a factor for equations for colligative properties, equal to the ratio of the number of actual particles present to the number of undissociated particles.

e. **False** – more correctly called Avogadro's constant, the Avogadro's number is the number of molecules of a gas present in 1 mol of the gas and is equal to 6.022×10^{23}.

4.27 Answers

a. **False.**
b. **True.**
c. **True.**
d. **False.**
e. **False.**

4.28 Answers

a. **True** – the visible range of EMRs is from c. 380 nm (violet) to c. 680 nm (red). Ultraviolet radiations are of three types: near UV or UV-A: 400–320 nm: UV-B: 320–290 nm: far UV or UV-C: 290–230 nm.
b. **True** – especially the short waves UV radiations.
c. **True** – the extreme UV radiations are absorbed by oxygen, which is converted into ozone in the process.
d. **True** – therefore lenses and prisms for use in ultraviolet light are made of quartz.
e. **True.**

4.29 Answers

a. **True** – helium still remains liquid at –269 °C (4 K).
b. **False** – upper airway obstruction because of its low density.
c. **True** – 'population inversion': maintenance of a higher proportion of the electrons of atoms or molecules of the lasing medium in the excited state compared with the ground state.
d. **False** – because of its higher thermal conductivity.
e. **False** – nitrogen under hyperbaric conditions is an anaesthetic. Therefore helium is used as a substitute because it needs an even higher pressure for helium to give it anaesthetic properties.

4.30 Answers

a. **False** – by fractional distillation of air. Brin process: conversion of barium oxide to barium peroxide at elevated temperature, followed by re-converting the barium peroxide to barium oxide, with release of the oxygen, at lower temperatures. It is now uneconomic and obsolete because of the feasibility of oxygen production by fractional distillation of air.
b. **True** – occurs in the vacuum-insulated evaporator.
c. **False** – J cylinders. There are no H cylinder sizes for medical gases in the UK.
d. **True.**
e. **True** – –118 °C.

4.31 Answers

a. **True** – any gas can be measured by the method of mass spectrometry.
b. **True.**
c. **False.**
d. **True.**
e. **False.**

4.32 Answers

a. **False** – by heating ammonium nitrate: $NH_4NO_3 \rightarrow N_2O + 2\,H_2O$.
b. **True** – N_2O: 36.4 °C; CO_2: 31.04 °C.
c. **False** – in this respect it differs from the higher oxides of nitrogen.
d. **True** – this is the basis of formation of entonox.
e. **False.**

4.33 Answers

a. **False** – it is an 'ideal' fluid that is regarded as incompressible.
b. **False** – it is the 'internal frictional forces' that gives it viscosity.
c. **True.**
d. **True** – shear stress: when a Newtonian fluid flows, due to the internal friction in the fluid, a tangential 'shear force' will exist between them as the fluid layers slide relative to one another. This shear force per unit area of fluid layer (F/A) is the 'shear stress'. Shear strain is the rate of shear produced between the different layers of fluid as a result of the velocity gradient between them.
e. **True.**

4.34 Answers

a. **True.**
b. **True.**
c. **True.**
d. **True.**
e. **False** – by measuring a pressure change.

4.35 Answers

a. **False** – Graham's Law: the rate of diffusion of a substance down its concentration gradient is inversely proportional to the square root of its molecular weight.
b. **True** – Henry's Law: the solubility of a gas in a liquid is directly proportional to its partial pressure.
c. **True** – Bunsen coefficient: the volume of gas, at 0 °C and standard atmospheric pressure, dissolved by unit volume of liquid when the partial pressure of the gas in contact is 1 standard atmospheric pressure.
d. **False.**
e. **False.**

4.36 Answers

a. **True.**
b. **False** – it is a spring-loaded valve.
c. **True.**
d. **False** – the Ruben valve, the predecessor of the Ambu valve, is a spring-loaded valve.
e. **False** – it is a spring-loaded valve.

4.37 Answers

a. **True.**
b. **True.**
c. **False.**
d. **True.**
e. **False.**

4.38 Answers

a. **False.**
b. **False.**
c. **False.**
d. **False.**
e. **True.**

4.39 Answers

a. **False** – it can occur with any gas.
b. **True** – used for the fractional distillation of air in the manufacture of oxygen.
c. **True.**
d. **False** – it is adiabatic compression that occurs at the Bodok seal interface on an anaesthetic machine.
e. **False** – results in a decrease in thermal energy viz. in a fall in temperature.

4.40 Answers

a. **True** – the competition between protons of different energy states for the magnetizing effect of the applied magnetic fields, leading to those with a lower energy state aligning themselves parallel to the magnetic field and those with a higher energy state aligning themselves antiparallel to the field.
b. **False** – population inversion is a phenomenon of the behaviour of lasers.
c. **False** – process by which attenuated ultrasound pulses from deeper interfaces in the body are amplified more than those originating closer to the ultrasound probe so as to magnify their signals.
d. **True** – ratio of the angular frequency ω (radians per second) of precessing protons to Bo (tesla), the external magnetic field.
e. **True** – decay of the vector of the transverse magnetism induced by the radiofrequency pulse when the latter is switched off.

4.41 Answers

a. **True** – it is expressed as joules per square metre, which is the same as 'newtons per metre', the conventional mode of expressing surface tension.
b. **False** – see **a** above.
c. **False** – because of the presence of hydrogen bonds.
d. **False.**
e. **False** – di-palmitoyl phosphatidyl choline (di-palmitoyl lecithin).

4.42 Answers

a. True – indeed it must be present for proper functioning of the soda lime.
b. True – the initial reaction is: $CO_2 + H_2O = H_2CO_3$; see **a** above.
c. True – for every molecule of CO_2 absorbed by soda lime, one molecule of water is used up and two molecules produced, therefore resulting in a net gain of one molecule of water.
d. False – water vapour does arise from patient exhalations. However, because of the interpositioning of an HMEF between patient end and Y-connection of the breathing tubes the patient's exhaled water vapour does not reach the soda lime.
e. False – decreases the likelihood of carbon monoxide formation.

4.43 Answers

a. True.
b. False – bore widens from bottom to top.
c. False.
d. False – need to be rendered antistatic to prevent the bobbin sticking to the side of the flowmeter tube.
e. False.

4.44 Answers

a. False – it is situated upstream of the pressure regulator at the cylinder–pin index block interface.
b. True.
c. True.
d. False – adiabatic compression.
e. True – but a seal of some sort is necessary so as to provide a gas-tight connection.

4.45 Answers

a. True – all oxygen cylinders, no matter their size, when full have a pressure of 137 bar.
b. True – empty weight: G cylinder: 35 kg; J cylinder: 70 kg.
c. False – about 10 times: E cylinder: 680 L; J cylinder: 6800 L.
d. False – pin index outlets for oxygen cylinders stop at size E.
e. False – ward cylinders: sizes F and G; bank cylinders: size J.

4.46 Answers

a. True – alternating blue and white quadrants.
b. False – size G.
c. True.
d. False – because the contents are normally entirely gaseous their contents can be determined by means of a pressure gauge.
e. True – D cylinders: 500 L; F cylinders: 2000 L.

4.47 Answers

a. **True.**
b. **False.**
c. **True.**
d. **True.**
e. **True** – but by the process of radiation only; heat transfer by conduction, convection and evaporation cannot occur in a vacuum.

4.48 Answers

a. **False.**
b. **False** – strictly speaking they are nonlinear so as to make allowance for the varying (zero) reference point.
c. **False.**
d. **False.**
e. **True.**

4.49 Answers

a. **False** – it decreases.
b. **True.**
c. **False** – at a certain temperature, the Curie temperature, a ferromagnetic material loses its ferromagnetic property and becomes paramagnetic.
d. **True.**
e. **False** – radioactive decay is independent of temperature.

4.50 Answers

a. **False** – by definition, a racemic mixture is a mixture of equal quantities of the dextro-rotatory and laevo-rotatory forms of an optically active compound and therefore has no optical activity of its own.
b. **False** – *cis–trans* isomerism may also be shown by a ring-structured compound.
c. **False.**
d. **True.**
e. **True** – therefore they have identical achiral properties such as melting point, boiling point, density, etc.

Practice paper 5

5.1   The following are SI units:

   a. Rem.
   b. Roentgen.
   c. Litre.
   d. Gray.
   e. Lux.

5.2   The following pairs have the same units of measurement:

   a. Work and energy.
   b. Pressure and strain.
   c. Electrical charge and quantum of electricity.
   d. Absolute temperature and thermodynamic temperature.
   e. Electrical resistance and electrical reactance.

5.3   The following are 'dimensionless entities':

   a. MAC.
   b. Specific gravity.
   c. Reflection coefficient.
   d. Specific heat capacity.
   e. Absorption coefficient (in relation to ultrasound imaging).

5.4   The following are dimensionless entities:

   a. Resistance (in relation to gas flow in conduits).
   b. Reactance (in relation to electricity).
   c. Reflectance (in relation to light).
   d. Elastance (in relation to the lung).
   e. Luminance (in relation to light).

5.5   The following refer to the same thing:

   a. Fundamental units and base units.
   b. Thermodynamic temperature and absolute temperature.
   c. Molar solution and normal solution.
   d. Electrical impedance and electrical resistance.
   e. Zero instability and alinearity (in relation to electronic monitoring equipment).

5.6   The variables in each of the following laws have a direct linear relationship:

   a. Charles' Law in relation to a gas.
   b. Gay-Lussac's Law in relation to a gas.
   c. Henry's Law in relation to solubility of a gas in a liquid.
   d. Graham's Law in relation to the rate of diffusion of a gas down its concentration gradient.
   e. Ohm's Law in respect of the relationship between resistance and current.

5.7 The following have an inverse relationship:

a. Voltage and amperage in a DC electrical circuit.
b. Reactance of a capacitor in an AC circuit and frequency of alternation of current in the circuit.
c. Reactance of an inductor in an AC circuit and frequency of alternation of current in the circuit.
d. Electrical conductivity of an insulator and temperature.
e. Energy of EMRs and the frequency of the radiation waves.

5.8 The following have the mathematical relationship $A \propto B^2$:

a. In turbulent flow the pressure gradient in the tube and the flow rate.
b. In laminar flow the flowrate and the cross-sectional area of the conduit.
c. The kinetic energy of a gas and the mean velocity of the gas molecules.
d. The heat generated by an electric current and the magnitude of the current.
e. The energy of EMRs and the amplitude of the waves.

5.9 The following laws of physics conform to the inverse square law in respect of the two quantities relating to each, as stated:

a. Boyle's Law in respect of volume and pressure.
b. Graham's Law of diffusion in respect of rate of diffusion of a substance down its concentration gradient and its molecular weight.
c. Stefan's Law in respect of the rate of emission of radiant energy by a black body emitter and its Kelvin temperature.
d. Van der Waals forces of attraction between gas molecules and the distance between the molecules.
e. Bouguer's Law in respect of the intensity of a light beam and the distance of propagation of the beam.

5.10 Each of the following relationships when graphically represented takes the form of an accelerating growth (i.e. positive) exponential:

a. Saturation vapour pressure of an halogenated inhalational anaesthetic agent and ambient temperature.
b. Haematocrit and blood viscosity.
c. Intra-alveolar pressure change during the inspiratory phase of IPPV with a constant pressure generator ventilator (such as the Manley MP 3 ventilator).
d. Relationship between electrical conductivity of a semiconductor and its temperature.
e. Relationship between the concentration of a substrate and the velocity of the corresponding enzyme-controlled reaction (Michaelis–Menton curve).

5.11 The 'half-life' in relation to processes:

a. Is a distinctive feature of exponential processes.
b. Is defined as 'half the time taken for all the activity to disappear'.
c. Is shorter than the 'time constant' of the process.
d. Is necessarily dependent on temperature.
e. Is characteristic for the decay of each radioactive isotope.

5.12   Reynolds number:

  a. Is a 'dimensionless entity'.
  b. Has an inverse relationship with fluid flow velocity.
  c. Is determined by both density and viscosity of the fluid.
  d. Is higher in the case of turbulent flow than with laminar flow.
  e. Other things being equal is less than 2000 for laminar flow.

5.13   The following phenomena exhibit time-related variation in a sinusoidal manner:

  a. Mains electricity voltage.
  b. Voltage in an isolated diathermy (electrosurgical unit) machine.
  c. Propagation of light in a laser beam.
  d. Energy discharge from an activated defibrillator capacitor.
  e. Vibration in a fluid-coupled transducer for invasive arterial BP monitoring.

5.14   The following refer to the same thing:

  a. Fundamental frequency and first harmonic.
  b. Ionic bond and electrovalent bond.
  c. Atomic mass and nucleon number.
  d. Collimation and coherence in respect of laser light.
  e. Remanence and coercivity in relation to MRI.

5.15   The basic physical principle that renders operational the following devices include the Bernoulli phenomenon and the Venturi effect:

  a. Anaesthetic machine variable orifice flowmeter tube.
  b. Sanders injector.
  c. Fixed performance oxygen mask.
  d. Pitot tube.
  e. Oxygen cut-off warning device on the anaesthetic machine.

5.16   The following statements are true:

  a. The Seebeck effect: generation of electrical resistance when two metal conductors of dissimilar materials are connected together at each end to form a circuit, which is proportional to the temperature difference of the two junctions.
  b. The Peltier effect: when an electric current is passed through a single junction between two dissimilar metals, heat is absorbed or liberated depending on the direction of the current.
  c. The Joule–Thomson effect: when a gas is subjected to sudden severe compression there is a rise in temperature of the gas.
  d. The Raman effect: when a beam of monochromatic light is passed through a medium the scattered radiation will have frequencies above and below the frequency of the incident beam.
  e. The Venturi effect: conversion of kinetic energy to potential energy when a fluid flowing along a conduit arrives at a constriction in the conduit.

5.17 The following are graded according to FCG (French catheter gauge):

a. Guedel oral airways.
b. Carlen double lumen tubes.
c. Ryle nasogastric tubes.
d. Tuohy epidural needles.
e. Whiteacre spinal needles.

5.18 The magnitude of the electric current in the following situations is of the order of milliamperes rather than amperes:

a. 'Interrogation current' of an REM (return electrode monitoring) diathermy plate.
b. 'Cannot let go' current of electrocution.
c. Diathermy current during a conventional TUR (transurethral resection) of prostate operation.
d. Standard current used for TENS (transcutaneous electrical nerve stimulation).
e. Tube current of a typical X-ray tube.

5.19 The following physical quantities are expressed in their respective units 'per metre' distance:

a. Surface tension.
b. Stress.
c. Permeability of free space (in relation to magnetism).
d. Permittivity of a vacuum (in relation to capacitance of a capacitor).
e. Strain.

5.20 The duration of the operational current energy stimulus of each of these devices is of the order of microseconds rather than milliseconds:

a. PNS (peripheral nerve stimulator) during Train-of-Four stimulation.
b. TENS (transcutaneous electrical nerve stimulation) machine.
c. Defibrillation current for correcting VF.
d. Discharge current during ECT.
e. Ultrasound pulse.

5.21 The following are associated with ultrasound imaging:

a. Piezo-electric effect.
b. Cavitation.
c. Acoustic mismatch.
d. Collimation.
e. Free induction decay.

5.22 The term luminescence encompasses the following phenomena:

a. Fluorescence.
b. Phosphorescence.
c. Thermoluminescence.
d. Scintillation.
e. Stimulated emission in relation to laser light.

5.23 In a hyperbaric chamber at 2 atmospheres pressure:

a. An anaesthetic rotameter will deliver a higher flow of gases than it actually indicates.
b. A 10% oxygen/90% nitrous oxide mixture will still be 'physiological'.
c. The same concentration setting on a Mark 4 isoflurane vaporizer will ensure the same level of anaesthesia as under normobaric conditions.
d. The orotracheal tube cuff will need less air for a gas-tight fit than under normobaric conditions.
e. An undrained pneumothorax will cause more respiratory embarrassment than under normobaric conditions.

5.24 When an electric current flows through a pure resistor in an AC circuit:

a. Voltage and current are in phase.
b. Impedance in the circuit is equal to resistance.
c. The circuit has reactance.
d. The circuit possesses inductance.
e. Ohm's Law correctly relates voltage, current and resistance.

5.25 The following statements are true:

a. All materials are by nature diamagnetic.
b. All bodies emit electromagnetic radiations at ambient temperature.
c. All gases will necessarily have solidified at temperatures near 0 kelvin.
d. All modes of heat loss from the human body are dependent on the presence of a 'downward' temperature gradient between the body and its surroundings.
e. All materials can be rendered electrically conductive provided a high enough potential difference can be maintained.

5.26 Sevoflurane can be assayed by the following methods of gas analysis:

a. Mass spectrometry.
b. Raman scattering.
c. Infrared gas analysis.
d. Paramagnetic analysis.
e. Piezo-electric method of gas analysis.

5.27 The presence of water vapour in a gas sample for analysis:

a. Can interfere with the accuracy of mass spectrometry.
b. Is likely to give erroneous carbon dioxide readings on infrared analysis.
c. Tends to give decreased values for levels of inhalational anaesthetic agents on infrared analysis.
d. Often creates problems with main stream gas analysers.
e. Can create problems with side stream analysers.

5.28 When laminar flow prevails in a fluid flow system:

a. The flow rate has a direct linear relationship with pressure gradient.
b. Reynolds number is less than 2000.
c. The viscosity of the fluid varies inversely with flow rate.
d. The fluid is essentially thixotropic in nature.
e. The density of the fluid is a material factor in determining fluid flow rate.

5.29 The gas flowmeter tubes of an anaesthetic machine:

a. Are based on a variable pressure differential, fixed orifice principle.
b. Have 'linear' calibrations.
c. Are no more accurate than to within a margin of about 10%.
d. Have tube bores which increase from bottom to top.
e. Need to be lined on their inside with metal for their accuracy of performance.

5.30 The following breathing attachments are regarded as more 'efficient' than the Magill attachment when used in spontaneous ventilation mode:

a. Bain co-axial attachment.
b. Bain non-co-axial attachment.
c. Parallel Lack attachment.
d. Waters to-and-fro attachment.
e. Ayre's T-piece attachment with Jackson Rees modification.

5.31 The 'infrared' thermometer when measuring tympanic membrane temperature:

a. Is based on the Stefan–Boltzmann principle.
b. Depends on the property of polarization of the sensor's constituent molecules.
c. Requires contact of sensor with the tympanic membrane for its correct performance.
d. Has a short response time.
e. May be taken as an accurate indicator of body core temperature.

5.32 The following are capable of being used as draw-over vaporizers:

a. Goldman vaporizer.
b. EMO (Epstein–Macintosh–Oxford) vaporizer.
c. Boyle bottle.
d. Fluotec Mark 2 vaporizer.
e. Desflurane (Mark 6) vaporizer.

5.33 The following statements are true with respect to mains electricity:

    a. It is transmitted through long distances at a potential in the kilovolt range.

    b. It has a peak phase voltage of about 240 V for ordinary domestic usage.

    c. Its frequency (of about 50 Hz) is the safest frequency with respect to the risk of electrocution.

    d. Its 'phase voltage' is higher than its 'line voltage'.

    e. It is usually 'earthed' at its substation.

5.34 The following refer to the same thing:

    a. Boyle's Law and Mariotte's Law.

    b. Boyle temperature and critical temperature.

    c. Beer's Law and Bouguer's Law.

    d. Avogadro's number and Avogadro's constant.

    e. Peltier effect and Seebeck effect.

5.35 A rise in temperature will lead to an increase in the following:

    a. Viscosity of a liquid.

    b. Solubility of a gas in a liquid.

    c. Density of a solid.

    d. Electrical conductivity of a semiconductor.

    e. Ferromagnetism of a ferromagnetic material.

5.36 The following describe the behaviour of gases when dissolving in liquids:

    a. Ostwald's coefficient.

    b. Joule effect.

    c. Raoult's Law.

    d. Bernoulli phenomenon.

    e. Coanda effect.

5.37 Compared with nitrous oxide, carbon dioxide has a higher:

    a. Molecular weight.

    b. Density.

    c. Critical temperature.

    d. Solubility in water.

    e. Viscosity.

5.38 The following statements are correct:

    a. All compounds contain London forces.

    b. All substances are diamagnetic by nature.

    c. All gases would have solidified at temperatures near 0 kelvin.

    d. All modes of heat transfer require an intervening medium.

    e. All stereo-isomers are necessarily enantiomers.

5.39 Other things being equal, protection from electrocution by operating theatre equipment is enhanced if:

a. The equipment is of Class II rather than Class I.
b. The equipment is DC powered rather than AC powered.
c. The operator of the equipment has a high skin impedance rather than low skin impedance.
d. The operator is using low resistance antistatic footwear rather than high resistance antistatic footwear.
e. The equipment is 'APG' rather than 'AP'.

5.40 The following processes involve an adiabatic change:

a. Fractional distillation of air.
b. Functioning of the cryoprobe.
c. Coanda effect.
d. Poynting effect.
e. Use of a zeolite for separating oxygen from air.

5.41 The fuel cell method of oxygen analysis:

a. Requires an 'external' potential difference.
b. Uses a platinum cathode.
c. Undergoes the same chemical reaction as does the Clark cell method.
d. Requires temperature control for its accuracy.
e. Is adversely affected by some inhalational anaesthetic agents.

5.42 Infrared radiations are absorbed by:

a. Oxygen.
b. Ozone.
c. Helium.
d. Nitric oxide.
e. Water vapour.

5.43 The following are desirable prerequisites for accuracy of electronic monitoring equipment:

a. High signal-to-noise ratio.
b. Low zero stability.
c. High frequency response.
d. Alinearity.
e. Ample reserve gain in system.

5.44 A size G oxygen cylinder:

a. Usually has a pin index outlet.
b. Contains twice the amount of oxygen as does a size F cylinder.
c. When full has the same gauge pressure as a size E cylinder.
d. Has an empty weight about twice the empty weight of a size F cylinder.
e. Is the cylinder size that is normally provided on the bottom of patient trolleys.

5.45 The presence of an inductor in the electrical circuit of a DC defibrillator:

   a. Is a necessary prerequisite for synchronized DC cardioconversion.
   b. Helps level out the current energy discharge through time.
   c. Helps to convert AC electricity to DC electricity within the circuit.
   d. Converts a monophasic current stimulus to a biphasic current stimulus.
   e. Can help reduce the risk of thermal injury to tissues.

5.46 The following have been recognized as affecting the accuracy of oxygen estimation by the method of paramagnetic analysis:

   a. Alterations in atmospheric pressure.
   b. Presence of water vapour in the gas sample.
   c. Nitric oxide.
   d. High flow rates of the sampled gases.
   e. Desflurane.

5.47 The Bourdon gauges on anaesthetic machines:

   a. Are accurate indicators of the contents of all cylinders on the machine.
   b. Have linear scales of graduations.
   c. Must according to ISO standards for the machine have their low pressure area in the 6 o'clock to 9 o'clock region of their dial face.
   d. Show a change in the cross-sectional configuration of their measuring tubes from elliptical to circular with decreasing cylinder pressure.
   e. Must according to ISO standards for the machine have their dial faces inclined 15 degrees backwards from the vertical.

5.48 The following oxides of nitrogen possess the property of paramagnetism:

   a. Nitrous oxide.
   b. Nitric oxide.
   c. Nitrogen dioxide.
   d. Nitrogen peroxide.
   e. Nitrogen pentoxide.

5.49 Pulse oximetry tends to give a falsely low SpO_2 reading in the presence of the following:

   a. Henna, a finger and toe stain, on skin and nails of fingers.
   b. Carboxyhaemoglobin in the blood.
   c. Dried blood on skin of sensing site.
   d. Ambient fluorescent lighting.
   e. Methylene blue dye in blood stream.

5.50 **An invasive blood pressure transducer system may be regarded as satisfactory if:**

a. It provides a frequency response up to the 10th harmonic of the pressure signal.
b. It is adjusted to 'critical damping'.
c. It has a damping factor adjusted to 1.0.
d. Its manometer has an undamped natural frequency considerably above that of the complete system.
e. Its fluid coupled transducer chamber has a larger volume rather than a smaller volume.

5.1 Answers

a. False – rem: 'roentgen equivalent man', the non-SI 'dose equivalent' unit of radiation. Its corresponding SI unit is the sievert.

b. False – Roentgen: non-SI unit of *exposure* and defines the intensity of radiations in terms of the ionization they produce in air and is equal to 2.58×10^{-4} coulombs per kilogram of air.

c. False – the corresponding SI unit is 10^{-3} cubic metres.

d. True – unit of absorbed dose; it is a measure of the energy transferred to a substance by radiations such as X-rays.

e. True – the SI unit of illuminance is equal to the illumination produced by a luminous flux of 1 lumen distributed uniformly over an area of 1 m^2.

5.2 Answers

a. True – the unit is the joule.

b. False – pressure and *stress* have the same units. Strain is a ratio and therefore is dimensionless.

c. True – the unit is the coulomb.

d. True – the unit is the kelvin.

e. True – they are both measured in ohms.

5.3 Answers

a. True – MAC (minimum alveolar concentration) at 1 atmosphere pressure of an inhalational anaesthetic agent that suppresses response to a painful stimulus in 50% of subjects. It is expressed as a percentage or a fraction.

b. True – now known as relative density, it is the ratio of the density (usually at 20 °C) of a substance to that of some reference substance, usually water.

c. True – the reflection coefficient is an indicator of the degree of capillary 'leakiness' to proteins and therefore is the ratio of the observed plasma colloid osmotic pressure to the theoretical osmotic pressure. It describes how a semipermeable membrane barrier excludes or 'reflects' plasma protein solutes as water moves across the barrier when driven by hydrostatic or osmotic pressure gradients. The reflection coefficient, σ, can range from 0 to 1. If the water, moving across the barrier, takes the solute completely along with it, then σ is zero. If the barrier totally prevents the solute from passing through it, then the solute exerts its full osmotic pressure and then σ is 1.

d. False – specific heat capacity: the amount of heat (in joules) required to raise the temperature of 1 kg of the substance by 1 K ($\text{J kg}^{-1} \text{ K}^{-1}$).

e. False – absorption coefficient: amount of absorption of the sound energy per unit distance travelled by the wave in a medium. It is stated for the particular frequency of the sound wave and is indicated in decibels per unit distance travelled (dB cm^{-1}).

5.4 Answers

a. **False** – resistance (to gas flow) is measured in cmH_2O pressure per unit flow rate.

b. **False** – reactance is the opposition to current flow in an AC circuit containing a capacitor and/or inductor. Its unit of measurement is the ohm.

c. **True** – reflectance: the amount of light energy reflected off a surface as a percentage of the light energy incident on the surface. It is therefore a ratio and thus dimensionless and is a factor that is relevant in surgical theatre lighting.

d. **False** – elastance (the opposite of compliance) is measured in cmH_2O pressure per unit volume of air.

e. **False** – luminance (photometric brightness) is the luminous intensity of a surface in a given direction per unit area of the surface as viewed from that direction. Units: candela per square metre.

5.5 Answers

a. **False** – the base units are the seven 'primary' units under the SI system: metre, kilogram, second, ampere, kelvin, candela and mole. Of these, the metre, kilogram and second are the three *fundamental* units and are the *dimensions* used to explain the whole of mechanics.

b. **True** – also known as Kelvin temperature.

c. **False** – a molar solution has 1 g mol of the solute in 1 L of solution. A normal solution has 1 g equivalent of solute in 1 L of solution.

d. **False** – they both indicate opposition to current flow in an electrical circuit. However, electrical resistance is only one form of impedance, the other being electrical *reactance*.

e. **False** – zero instability refers to the inability of a monitoring system to maintain a zero reading on the display when the input signal is zero. Alinearity is the inability to maintain equal degrees of amplification of the output signal for equal degrees of the input signal over the whole range of signal strengths.

5.6 Answers

a. **True** – Charles' Law: the volume of a fixed mass of gas at constant pressure varies directly with its thermodynamic temperature.

b. **True** – Gay-Lussac's Law: the pressure of a fixed mass of gas at constant volume varies directly with its thermodynamic temperature.

c. **True** – Henry's Law: the concentration of a solute gas in a solution is directly proportional to the partial pressure of that gas above the solution. Strictly speaking, Henry's Law holds good only for the behaviour of gases dissolving in liquids when concentrations and partial pressures are reasonable low. As concentrations and partial pressures increase, deviations from the law become marked; cf. the behaviour of gases in relation to the gas laws. But for practical purposes the relationship may be regarded as linear.

d. **False** – Graham's Law: the rate of diffusion of a gas down its concentration gradient is *inversely* proportional to the *square root* of its molecular weight:

$$D \propto \frac{1}{\sqrt{MW}}.$$

e. **False** – resistance and current have an inverse relationship when the voltage is constant: $V = iR$; therefore $i \propto \frac{1}{R}$.

5.7 Answers

a. **False** – the relationship is linear; see **5.6e**.

b. **True** – the relationship is: $X_c = \frac{1}{2\pi fC}$, where X_c is the capacitance reactance, f is the frequency of the alternating current and C is the capacitance of the capacitor in farads.

c. **False** – the relationship is direct: $X_L = 2\pi fL$, where X_L is the inductor reactance, f is the frequency of alternating current, and L is the value of the inductance in henrys.

d. **False** – the electrical conductivity of an insulator increases with temperature (but the change is not linear). Note: it appears a contradiction to speak of the electrical conductivity of an insulator, because by definition an insulator prevents the passage of electricity. However, there is no such thing as a perfect insulator; given a high enough voltage an insulator will allow the passage of electricity through it.

e. **False** – the higher the frequency of EMRs, the higher their energy. The relationship is direct and linear: $E = hf$, where E is in joules, f is in hertz and h is the Planck constant: 6.6262×10^{-34} J s.

5.8 Answers

a. **True** – $\dot{Q} \propto \sqrt{P}$; therefore, $P \propto \dot{Q}^2$.

b. **True** – in laminar flow $\dot{Q} \propto r^4$; therefore, $\dot{Q} \propto$ cross-sectional area^2.

c. **True** – because kinetic energy is equal to $\frac{1}{2}mv^2$.

d. **True** – heat (joules) = volts × current × time. Since volts = current × resistance, heat = current^2 × resistance × time. Therefore, heat $\propto$ current^2.

e. **True**.

5.9 Answers

a. False – Boyle's Law is an example of the 'Inverse' Law: $A \propto \frac{1}{B}$, not of the inverse square law: $A \propto \frac{1}{B^2}$.

b. True – Graham's Law: the rate of diffusion of a substance down its concentration gradient is inversely proportional to the square root of its molecular weight. Therefore, $D \propto \frac{1}{\sqrt{MW}}$. Squaring both sides gives: $D^2 \propto \frac{1}{MW}$. Therefore, $MW \propto \frac{1}{D^2}$.

c. False – rate of emission of energy by a black body radiator is directly proportional to the fourth power of its Kelvin temperature: $E \propto T^4$.

d. False – van der Waals forces of attraction between gas molecules are inversely proportional to the seventh power of the distance between them: $F \propto \frac{1}{D^7}$.

e. True – Bouguer's Law is the same as Lambert's Law.

5.10 Answers

a. True.

b. True.

c. False – a decelerating growth exponential.

d. True – it increases exponentially.

e. False – a decelerating growth exponential.

5.11 Answers

a. True.

b. False – it is the 'time taken for half the activity to disappear', i.e. for the activity to fall to one-half of its initial value. Note: since in an exponential process the activity cannot mathematically come to an end, i.e. it is an infinite process, then half the time taken for it must also be infinite.

c. True – equal to 69.3% of the time constant.

d. False – it is temperature dependent in the case of biological processes, but independent of temperature in most other processes, e.g. in the case of radioactive decay.

e. True.

5.12 Answers

a. True – because the dimensions of the variables that form the numerator are the same as those of the denominator, and therefore cancel each other out.

b. False – directly proportional to fluid flow velocity.

c. True.

d. True.

e. True.

Note: Reynolds number: $= \frac{V\rho l}{\eta}$, where v is velocity of flow, ρ is density of fluid, l is length of conduit and η is viscosity of fluid.

5.13 Answers

a. True – at a frequency of 50 Hz.
b. True – at a frequency of 3.5 MHz. The fact that the machine is 'isolated' is irrelevant; it is a red herring!
c. True – the frequency is that of the particular wavelength. The fact that it is laser light and not ordinary light is irrelevant.
d. False – defibrillators discharge DC electricity. So there cannot be a time-related sinusoidal variation of the electrical quantities.
e. True.

5.14 Answers

a. True.
b. True.
c. True – the atomic mass (formerly known as atomic weight) of an element is equal to the number of nucleons (i.e. neutrons and protons) present in its atoms.
d. False – collimation: the absence of divergence of the light beam in relation to distance of propagation. Coherence: all the waves are in phase, with the result that their energies are additive. It is these two properties that impart intense brightness to a laser light beam.
e. False – remanence: the magnetic intensity remaining in a ferromagnetic core when the magnetizing force has been reduced to zero. Coercivity: the further magnetizing force required to reduce the magnetic flux density to zero.

5.15 Answers

a. False.
b. True.
c. True.
d. False.
e. False.

5.16 Answers

a. False – the result is the generation of an EMF.
b. True.
c. False – the *lowering* of temperature resulting from *decompression* is the Joule–Thomson effect.
d. True.
e. False – the conversion is of potential energy to kinetic energy, and it is known as the Bernoulli phenomenon. The Venturi effect is the entrainment of air (or liquid) as a result of the lowering of pressure resulting from the decrease in potential energy.

5.17 Answers

a. False – Guedel airways have an 'arbitrary' numbering.
b. True – their numbers are 35, 37, 39 and 41.
c. True.
d. False – numbered according to SWG.
e. False – numbered according to SWG.

Note: FCG stands for 'French catheter gauge' and is a measure of the external circumference in millimetres of the device. SWG, 'steel wire gauge', denotes the number of wires of the same diameter as the device that could be accommodated within a standard lumen. It has no units and, furthermore, the larger the size the smaller the device. SWG sizes are normally applied to needles and epidural catheters. FCG size is applied to tracheostomy tubes, stomach tubes, chest drain tubes, suction catheters and Robertshaw double lumen tubes and quadruple lumen central venous catheters. Guedel airways have 'arbitrary' numbering, and orotracheal tubes, the odd ones out, are designated by their internal diameter in millimetres.

5.18 Answers

a. True – 2 mA current (at a frequency of 140 kHz).
b. True – c. 15–20 mA.
c. False – about 1–2 A.
d. True – up to 50 mA.
e. True – 200–500 mA. Note: this must be distinguished from the 'filament heating current', which is of the order of 5–10 A.

5.19 Answers

a. True – measured in newtons per metre, but can also be stated as 'joules per square metre'.
b. False – stress has the same units as pressure: newtons per square metre.
c. True – a measure of the ease with which a material is magnetized and is measured in henrys per metre.
d. True – measure of the ability of a material to store electric energy and is measured in farads per metre.
e. False – strain is a ratio and is therefore dimensionless.

5.20 Answers

a. True – c. 200–300 μs.
b. True – 100–500 μs.
c. False – 3–5 ms.
d. False – 0.5–4.0 ms.
e. True – 10 μs.

5.21 Answers

a. True – the ultrasound waves are formed by the action of a high frequency (3–5 MHz) electric current on a piezo-electric crystal.

b. True – sudden collapse of gas-filled cavities in tissues following the high pressure resulting from the ultrasound wave.

c. True – difference in specific acoustic impedance of two media will lead to 'acoustic mismatch' at the media interface. The outcome of this is that most of the ultrasound wave is likely to be reflected at the interface.

d. False – collimation: nondivergence of a wave, a particular property of laser light beams.

e. False – free induction decay is a feature of MRI scanning.

5.22 Answers

a. True.
b. True.
c. True.
d. True.
e. True.

Note: *luminescence*: emission of light by a substance as a result of a process that does not involve a rise in temperature (e.g. fluorescent 'strip' light); cf. *incandescence*: emission of light as a result of a rise in temperature (e.g. ordinary electric light bulb).

5.23 Answers

a. True.
b. True.
c. True.
d. False – it will need more air.
e. True – because the air in the pneumothorax will be at twice the usual pressure and therefore will cause double the respiratory embarrassment.

5.24 Answers

a. True.
b. True – impedance in relation to electricity is a generic term for opposition to passage of electric current in a circuit and includes both *resistance* (opposition to current flow in a resistor) and *reactance* (opposition to current flow in a capacitor and/or inductor). If, therefore, there is only a pure resistor in the circuit, the opposition to current flow is solely in the form of resistance.

c. False – reactance is only present in an AC circuit which has capacitance and/or inductance; see **b** above.

d. False – see c above.

e. True.

5.25 Answers

a. True.

b. True – all bodies will emit EMRs provided their temperatures are above 0 K.

c. False – helium will still remain liquid at 4 K and therefore it is used as a supercoolant in the MRI scanner.

d. False – evaporation (by respiration or perspiration) can occur against a temperature gradient.

e. True – in other words there is no such thing as a 'perfect insulator'; see **5.7d**.

5.26 Answers

a. True.

b. True.

c. True.

d. False.

e. True.

5.27 Answers

a. True – if it is a 'rogue gas', i.e. if the appliance is not designed to measure it.

b. True – because water absorbs infrared radiations.

c. False – gives increased values.

d. False – seldom do.

e. True.

5.28 Answers

a. True.

b. True.

c. False – the flow rate of a fluid is determined by, among other things, its viscosity, and the relationship is inverse in accordance with the Hagen–Poiseuille equation. But the viscosity for any particular fluid under laminar flow conditions is constant and does not vary with varying fluid flow rate.

d. False – a thixotropic fluid is one whose viscosity varies inversely with the flow rate. Blood is a thixotropic fluid.

e. False.

5.29 Answers

a. False – variable orifice–constant pressure differential principle.

b. False – the markings are 'logarithmoid' in gradation.

c. False – accurate to within 2–5%.

d. True.

e. True – are lined with tin or aluminium oxide to render them antistatic.

5.30 Answers

a. **False.**
b. **False.**
c. **True.**
d. **False** – unless it incorporates a provision for soda lime absorption.
e. **False.**

Note: the 'efficiency' of a breathing attachment for spontaneous ventilation is gauged by determining the ratio of the fresh gas flow rate to minute volume required to maintain normocapnia. If the ratio is less than 1 the attachment is regarded as 'more efficient'; if more than 1, 'less efficient'.

5.31 Answers

a. **True** – Stefan–Boltzmann principle; the total energy radiated per unit surface area of a black body radiator is proportional to the fourth power of its Kelvin temperature: $E \propto T^4$.
b. **False.**
c. **False** – because the thermometer 'reads' EMR radiations, which are transmissible from the tympanic membrane to the sensor of the thermometer, there is no need for physical contact between sensor and tympanic membrane.
d. **True.**
e. **True** – because it indicates the temperature of the tympanic membrane, which is supplied by a branch of the internal carotid artery, which provides blood to the core of the brain.

5.32 Answers

a. **True.**
b. **True.**
c. **False.**
d. **True** – the Mark 2 (halothane) vaporizer was the first TEC vaporizer to be clinically used and had a very low internal resistance, and therefore could be used as a draw-over vaporizer, although it was rarely so used.
e. **False.**

5.33 Answers

a. **True** – it is generated at about 25 000 V and transmitted at a voltage varying between 125 000 and 400 000 V.
b. **False** – 240 is the RMS (root mean square) voltage. The mains electricity is at a peak voltage of 339 V.
c. **False** – it is the least safe frequency because electricity at a frequency of 50 Hz has the lowest threshold for causing VF.
d. **False** – mains electricity is 'tri-phasic', i.e. there are three simultaneously produced supplies available to the consumer. 'Phase' voltage refers to the voltage when a single supply is in use and has an RMS voltage of 240 V. A 'line voltage' results when two such supplies provide the electrical energy. Their combined voltage is not 480 (i.e. 240 × 2) but 419 (i.e 240 × $\sqrt{3}$) because one of them is 'out of phase' by 120 degrees in relation to the other.
e. **True** – this is by means of a 'functional earth', the purpose of which is to protect the system.

5.34 Answers

a. True – Edme Mariotte (1620–1684), a founder member of the French Academy of Science, discovered the law independently in 1676. Robert Boyle discovered it in 1662.

b. False – 'critical temperature': the temperature above which a gas cannot be liquefied by pressure alone. Boyle temperature: the temperature at which a gas most closely approximates to an ideal gas.

c. False – Bouguer's Law is the same as Lambert's Law, not Beer's Law. Pierre Bouguer (1698–1758), the French physicist, described the same phenomenon as Johann Heinrich Lambert (1728–1777): the intensity of a beam of light is inversely proportional to the square of its distance from its source.

d. True – the number of molecules of a substance present in 1 mol of the substance: 6.022×10^{23}.

e. False – the two are the opposites of each other. Seebeck effect (after Thomas Seebeck [1770–1831]): generation of an EMF in a circuit containing two different metals (or semiconductors) when the two junctions of the metals are maintained at two different temperatures. Peltier effect (after Jean Peltier [1785–1845]): change in temperature resulting at a junction between two dissimilar metals (or semiconductors) on passage of an electric current through the junction.

5.35 Answers

a. False – the viscosity of a liquid decreases with temperature, that of a gas increases.

b. False.

c. False – the density decreases because the volume increases while the mass remains the same.

d. True – conductors lower their conductivity with a rise in temperature, semiconductors and insulators increase their conductivity.

e. False – in fact at a certain temperature, known as the Curie temperature, a ferromagnetic material loses that property and becomes only paramagnetic.

5.36 Answers

a. True – Ostwald's solubility coefficient: volume of gas dissolved in unit volume of liquid at the particular temperature and pressure of the solution.

b. False – Joule effect: liberation of heat from a conductor when an electric current flows in it.

c. True – Raoult's Law: the partial vapour pressure of a solvent is proportional to the mole fraction of the solvent in the particular solution.

d. False – Bernoulli phenomenon: at any point in a pipe through which a fluid is flowing the sum of the kinetic energy and potential energy of a given mass of the fluid is a constant.

e. False – Coanda effect (or wall-attachment effect): the tendency of a moving fluid to attach itself to a surface and flow along it. As a fluid moves across a surface a certain amount of friction occurs between the fluid and the surface, which tends to slow the moving fluid. This resistance to the flow of the fluid pulls the fluid towards the surface, causing it to stick to the surface. The phenomenon was observed in 1930 by Henri Coanda (1886–1972).

5.37 Answers

a. False – they both have the same molecular weight, viz. 44.

b. False – same (at 15 °C and 1 bar pressure): the density is the same, viz. 1.85 kg/m³ (because their molecular weights are the same).

c. False – CO_2: 31 °C; N_2O: 36.4 °C.

d. True – solubility in water: Ostwald's coefficient at 1 bar and 25 °C: CO_2: 0.870; N_2O: 0.838.

e. True – the viscosity is marginally higher (at 25 °C): CO_2: 0.0150 mPa s; N_2O: 0.0147 mPa s.

5.38 Answers

a. True.

b. True.

c. False – helium still remains liquid at 4 K, hence its use as a supercoolant in the MRI scanner.

d. False – heat transfer by radiation can occur in a vacuum.

e. False – may be diastereomers.

5.39 Answers

a. True – Class II equipment is 'double insulated'.

b. True – a higher current energy is required with DC equipment compared with AC equipment.

c. True – a high impedance will reduce the current passing through the body.

d. False – high resistance footwear will reduce the current passing through the body to the ground.

e. False – AP and APG are not modes of categorization of equipment with respect to their potential to cause electrocution. They are modes of classification of 'anaesthetic proof' equipment based on the ignition energy required to ignite the most flammable mixture of ether and carrier gas. AP ('anaesthetic proof') standard equipment can be used at a distance between 5 and 25 cm from such an inflammable anaesthetic gas mixture escaping from an anaesthetic breathing attachment. APG ('anaesthetic proof gas') is a more stringent standard and is based on the ignition energy required to ignite the most flammable mixture of ether and *oxygen*. The equipment can be used within 5 cm of a flammable gas mixture.

5.40 Answers

a. True – adiabatic expansion.

b. True – adiabatic expansion.

c. False.

d. False.

e. False.

5.41 Answers

a. False – it is the Clark cell method that requires an 'external' potential difference; the fuel cell generates its own potential difference.

b. False – lead anode and gold cathode. Clark cell: Ag/AgCl anode and platinum cathode.

c. True – $O_2 + 4e + 2H_2O = 4OH^-$.

d. True – so does the Clark cell.

e. True – affected by nitrous oxide. The Clark cell is affected by halothane.

5.42 Answers

a. False.

b. False.

c. False.

d. True.

e. True.

Note: infrared radiations are absorbed by gases if they have two or more dissimilar atoms in their molecules.

5.43 Answers

a. True.

b. False.

c. True.

d. False.

e. True.

5.44 Answers

a. False – pin index outlets for oxygen cylinders only apply to cylinders C, D and E.

b. False – F cylinder: 1360 L; G cylinder: 3400 L.

c. True – all oxygen cylinders, no matter their size, have a 'full' pressure of 137 bar.

d. False – approximate empty weights of oxygen cylinders in kilograms: D: 3.5; E: 5.4; F: 14.5; G: 35; J: 70.

e. False – trolleys normally have size F oxygen cylinders. Size G cylinders are the common 'upstanding' cylinders found on wards.

5.45 Answers

a. False – an inductor helps level out the energy discharge from the capacitor over time. Its presence will improve the efficiency of the capacitor discharge and therefore the chances of successful defibrillation. However, it is not a necessary prerequisite for the functioning of the defibrillator.

b. True – see **a** above.

c. False – AC–DC conversion is done by a rectifier (diode).

d. False.

e. True – by levelling out the current energy level over time.

5.46 Answers

a. **True.**
b. **True.**
c. **True** – because nitric oxide is a paramagnetic gas.
d. **False.**
e. **True** – a gas mixture containing desflurane has been known to interfere with the accuracy of paramagnetic analysers.

5.47 Answers

a. **False** – only those cylinders whose contents are entirely gaseous.
b. **True** – they are of equal magnitude.
c. **True.**
d. **False** – from circular to elliptical with decreasing pressure.
e. **True.**

5.48 Answers

a. **False.**
b. **True.**
c. **True.**
d. **False.**
e. **False.**

5.49 Answers

a. **True.**
b. **False** – leads invariably to a near normal reading irrespective of the actual SpO_2 level.
c. **False** – no effect.
d. **False** – can falsely elevate reading especially if the flicker frequency of the light is close to a harmonic of the diode sensitivity frequency.
e. **True** – lowers readings in a dose-related manner.

5.50 Answers

a. **True.**
b. **False** – optimal damping.
c. **False** – adjusted to c. 0.7.
d. **True.**
e. **False** – smaller volume.

Appendix 1: Isomerism

Isomers are substances that have the same *elemental composition* but differ in their *atomic alignments*. There are two types:

1. *structural* (or constitutional) isomers; and
2. *stereo-isomers* (or configurational isomers).

Structural isomers differ from each other in their *connectivity*, i.e. the order in which the different atoms are connected to each other. Connectivity differences may be due to: (i) different carbon skeletons:

$$CH_3-CH_2-CH_2-CH_3 \qquad\qquad CH_3-CH-CH_3$$
$$\qquad\qquad\qquad\qquad\qquad\qquad\qquad\quad |$$
$$\qquad\qquad\qquad\qquad\qquad\qquad\qquad\; CH_3$$

       Butane   2-Methyl propane

(ii) the same carbon skeleton but different placement of functional groups:

```
      F F   F                    F H   F
      | |   |                    | |   |
   H–C–C–O–C–H              F–C–C–O–C–H
      | |   |                    | |   |
     Cl F   F                    F Cl  F
    Enflurane                   Isoflurane
```

and (iii) different carbon skeletons *and* different placement of functional groups:

$$CH_3-CH_2-OH \qquad\qquad\qquad CH_3-O-CH_3$$

               Ethanol   Dimethyl ether

One particular form of structural isomerism is *tautomerism*, also known as *dynamic isomerism*. In keto–enol tautomerism a compound containing a $-CH_2-CO-$ group (keto form) is in equilibrium with a $-CH - C-(OH)$ group (enol form), as the result of migration of an H atom between a carbon atom and the oxygen of an adjacent carbon, as in pentobarbitone, or a sulphur atom, as in thiopentone. In latter case, it is the enol to keto change on intravenous injection, resulting from a change in environmental pH, which gives thiopentone its pharmacological activity.

Lactam–lactim tautomerism is a similar form of dynamic isomerism. Lactam is an organic compound in ring form in which $-NH-CO-$ forms part of the ring; whereas lactim is an organic compound in ring form in which $-N=C(OH)-$ forms part of the ring.

$$\gamma \quad \beta \quad \alpha$$

$$NH_2-CH_2-CH_2-CH_2-COOH$$

Gamma amino butyric acid (GABA)

$$CH_2-CH_2-C=O$$
$$\begin{array}{cc} | & | \\ CH_2 & ——NH \end{array}$$

γ-lactam ring

$$CH_2-CH_2-C-OH$$
$$\begin{array}{cc} | & \nearrow\nearrow \\ CH_2 & —N \end{array}$$

γ-lactim ring

Stereo-isomers have the same atomic *connectivity,* i.e. the order in which the different atoms are connected to each other, but differ in their *configurations,* i.e. the spatial disposition of the various substituents. Stereo-isomers may be classified in different ways. A common classification is into:

1. enantiomers, which are nonsuperimposable mirror images of each other; and
2. diastereomers, which are not mirror images of each other.

Two compounds constitute a pair of enantiomers if:

1. the molecules of the two compounds are mirror images of each other; and
2. the molecules of the two compounds are nonsuperimposable on each other.

A molecule that is nonsuperimposable on its mirror image molecule is said to be chiral or to possess chirality, 'handedness'.

A pair of enantiomers is possible only when a compound contains a tetrahedral stereocentre, i.e. it has an atom, invariably a carbon atom, with four different substituents. A stereocentre is an atom in a compound bearing substituents of such identity that a hypothetical exchange of the positions of any two substituents would convert one stereo-isomer into another stereo-isomer.

Enantiomers may be classified as D- and L-forms. This system is simple and easy to understand, but is limited because of the lack of three-dimensional perspective. A more recent system is the *R/S* system. The D/L system is based on the Fischer projection and relates the structure of the compound to a reference molecule, viz. glyceraldehyde. The structure of the compound is represented in two-dimensional form in which the horizontal bonds are deemed to extend in front of the plane of the paper and the vertical bonds behind the plane of the paper. The structure of glyceraldehyde is written with the asymmetric carbon atom in the centre, the –CHO group at the top and the CH_2OH at the bottom. If the H is attached to the left of the carbon and the –OH to the right, the molecule is D-glyceraldehyde. If the –OH is placed to the left of the carbon, the molecule is L-glyceraldehyde.

$$\begin{array}{c} CHO \\ | \\ H-C-OH \\ | \\ CH_2OH \end{array} \qquad\qquad \begin{array}{c} CHO \\ | \\ HO-C-H \\ | \\ CH_2OH \end{array}$$

D-glyceraldehyde   L-glyceraldehyde

It is important to bear in mind that the prefixes D- and L- denote an 'arbitrary' convention and do not stand for dextro-rotatory and laevo-rotatory (*d*- and *l*-). In fact a D-compound could be laevorotatory (*l*-form) and an L-compound dextro-rotatory (*d*-form).

D- and L-isomerism is important in human biology. For instance, the 'essential' amino acids in the body are all L-amino acids, and it is only the D-forms of sugars that are normally absorbed in the gut.

The *R/S* nomenclature, also known as the Cahn–Ingold–Prelog nomenclature, is a convention based on priority of order of attachment of substituent groups to the chiral carbon atom, hydrogen having the lowest priority, and the molecule being viewed 'end on' with the group of lowest priority behind the chiral atom. If the clockwise arrangement of the other three groups is in descending priority, the compound is an *R*-compound; if the descending priority is anticlockwise, it is an *S*-compound.

Enantiomers differ from achiral compounds in one physical property – optical activity, and one chemical property – chiral recognition. The two enantiomers of a pair of enantiomers rotate the plane of plane-polarized light in opposite directions but by the same number of degrees. They are therefore named *dextro-rotatory* (*d*-form) and *laevo-rotatory* (*l*- form) or (+) and (–), respectively.

It is important to note the significance of the different nomenclatures: *R* and *S*, D and L, *d* and *l*, and (+) and (–). The first two relate to configuration, which is based on a prescribed convention. The *d* and *l* [and (+) and (–)] are based on optical rotation and therefore on empirical evidence relating to the actual behaviour of compounds with respect to plane-polarized light rotation.

Diastereomers are usually optically active but, unlike enantiomers, have specific rotations that usually differ in their numerical value, i.e. the degree of rotation, and may have the same or the opposite direction of rotation. Furthermore, unlike enantiomers, diastereomers also differ in other physical properties such as melting point, boiling point and solubility.

One particular type of diastereomerism is *cis–trans* isomerism or geometric isomerism. In this type of isomerism the atomic connectivity of the substituents of the isomers is the same but their spatial orientation is different. For *cis–trans* isomerism to exist the compound must have two asymmetric carbon atoms either separated by a double bond, if the compound is a 'straight chain' compound, or part of a ring structure, if the carbon atoms are separated by only a single bond.

Cis–trans isomerism is of significant biological importance, e.g. in vision. The rod and cone cells of the retina contain rhodopsin, a molecular complex of opsin and *cis*-11-retinal. When light strikes a molecule of *cis*-11-retinal, the photoenergy breaks one of the bonds of the carbon–carbon double bond, the atoms rotate and the cis-11-retinal is isomerized to *trans*-11-retinal, with a change in shape of the retinal. This allows the retinal to dissociate from the opsin moiety resulting in the transmission of an electrical signal to the optic nerve. Subsquent re-conversion of the *trans* form to the *cis* form by the enzyme retinal isomerase restores the status quo.

Appendix 2: SI units

Base quantities and units

Physical quantity	Unit	Symbol
Length	metre	m
Mass	kilogram	kg
Time	second	s
Electric current	ampere	A
Thermodynamic temperature	kelvin	K
Intensity of illumination	candela	cd
Amount of substance	mole	mol

The three fundamental quantites and units are mass (kilogram), length (metre) and time (second).

Supplementary quantities and units are plane angle (radian) and solid angle (steradian).

Derived units

Physical quantity	Unit	Symbol
Frequency	hertz	Hz
Force	newton	N
Pressure	pascal	Pa
Work, energy, quantity of heat	joule	J
Power	watt	W
Quantity of electricity	coulomb	C
Electrical potential	volt	V
Electrical resistance	ohm	Ω
Electrical capacitance	farad	F
Magnetic flux	weber	Wb
Magnetic flux density	tesla	T
Inductance	henry	H
Radioactivity	becquerel	Bq
Unit of absorbed dose	gray	Gy
Unit of dose equivalent	sievert	Sv

Commonly used non-SI units
Pressure – millimetre mercury (mmHg), bar
Length – angstrom (Å)
Volume – litre (L)

SI units

The SI Units (Système International d'Unitès) came into force in 1960. Prior to this, there was the Imperial System of measurement, as well as a Metric system, the latter based on the centimetre, gram and second (also known as the cgs system). The purpose of the SI Units was:

- To have a universal system of measurement so that everyone 'spoke the same mathematical language'.
- To have a decimal system so that fractions and multiples of units would change by a factor of 10.
- To adopt the metric (French) system for at least the common units of measurement.

There are seven **base quantities** in the SI nomenclature with their corresponding **units**:

Mass	Kilogram	How massive is it?
Length	Metre	What is its size?
Time	Second	How does it vary over time?
Electric current	Ampere	How much electric current flows through it?
Thermodynamic temperature	Kelvin	How hot is it?
Intensity of illumination	Candela	How bright is it?
Amount of substance	Mole	How many elementary particles does it contain?

Definitions of the units

Mass in kilograms: a mass equal to that of the international prototype kilogram, a platinum-iridium cylinder in the International Bureau of Weights and Measures at Sevres, France.

Length in metres: the metre was first taken to be equal to one ten millionth of the earth's meridian quadrant passing through Paris, in 1791. In 1793, it was defined by reference to a length of platinum. In 1958, the metre was defined by reference to the radiations emanating from krypton in a vacuum, and in 1967, by reference to the distance travelled by light in a vacuum in $1/299\,792\,458$ths of a second. This last definition was adopted by the General Conference on Weights and Measures in October 1983.

Time in seconds: duration corresponding to a number of periods of the radiations in caesium-133.

Electric current in amperes: that constant current which, if maintained in two parallel straight conductors of infinite length, of negligible cross-section and placed 1 metre apart in a vacuum, would produce between them a force of 2×10^{-7} newtons per metre of length.

Thermodynamic temperature in kelvin: the fraction $1/273.16$ of the thermodynamic temperature of the triple point of water.

Intensity of illumination in candela: the luminous intensity, in the perpendicular direction of a surface of $1/600\,000$ square metres of a black body radiator at the temperature of freezing platinum (1773 °C) under a pressure of 101 325 newtons per square metre (1 bar).

Amount of substance in moles: that amount of substance of a system which contains as many elementary entities as there are atoms in 0.012 kilograms of carbon-12. Note that while mass is defined with respect to the kilogram, the amount of substance is defined as a mole, not kilomole.

Oddities

One reason for the institution of the SI Units was the need to move away from actual physical entities when defining base quantities and units. However, one unit is still defined by reference to an actual physical entity viz. the kilogram. It is a unit of mass equal to the mass of the international prototype kilogram, a platinum-iridium cylinder preserved at the International Bureau of Weights and Measures at Sevres, France. There are moves to re-define the kilogram by reference to the mass of a certain number of atoms of an element such as silicon, but this has not been formally ratified.

Temperature is the only quantity that is not 'extensive', i.e. it does not contain 'positive fiduciary marks'. An extensive property is a property whose magnitude depends on the amount of the substance present in a given thermodynamic state.

Time is the only quantity that is not 'decimalized'; the conversion of seconds to minutes and hours to days does not involve conversion factors of 10 or its multiples.

Although the unit of mass is the kilogram, the unit of quantity of substance is the mole, not the kilomole.

The definitions of some units presuppose the existence of other units, both base and derived. For example, the ampere is defined by reference to the metre as well as the unit of force, the newton. The definition of the candela is by reference to the unit of temperature as well as the square metre.

Apart from the **base** units and the **derived** units, there are also two **supplementary** units, the radian (unit of two-dimensional or plane angle) and the steradian (unit of three-dimensional or solid angle). Three of the base units – metre, kilogram and second – are also known as **fundamental** units. They are also referred to as 'dimensions', and all the quantities in mechanics can be expressed in terms of these three units. Furthermore, the dimensions on the two sides of any physical equation must be the same; otherwise the equation is not scientifically valid.

Finally, there are also **non-SI** units. Some of these are still used in science and therefore relevant to medical practice. They include the millimetre of mercury (mmHg), bar, angstrom and centimetre of water (cm H_2O).

For reasons of clarity and to avoid ambiguity, there are certain conventions for the manner of denoting SI units. When abbreviated, no punctuation marks shall be used. For example:

- 'Kilogram' shall be written '1 kg ', not '1 kg.', i.e. with a dot after the abbreviation.
- Abbreviations shall have no plural forms, e.g. '200 metres' shall be written '200 m', not '200 ms'. 'ms' in fact stands for 'millisecond'.

When written in full, the names of units shall not commence with a capital (upper case) letter, unless it is at the beginning of a sentence. However, eponymous units, i.e. those named after a person, when in abbreviated form shall be shown by a capital letter (e.g. 'N' for newton) and, when there is more than one letter in the abbreviation, the first letter alone shall be upper case (e.g. kPa for kilopascals, Hz for hertz). Capital letters are also used for certain unit multiples, e.g. GBq for gigabecquerels, MHz for megahertz;

No 'degree' sign shall be used for the kelvin scale; therefore, it is '230 kelvin', not '230 ° kelvin', because the scale is an absolute scale and there are no 'degrees' in it;

Mathematical indicial notation shall be used, not the solidus notation (the / sign]. So 'metres per second' should be written as m s^{-1}, not 'm/s'.

No multiplication signs should be used to denote the product of two (or more) units, but the units shall be separated by a space, e.g. metre × seconds shall be written as m s, not m × s. The space is important because ms is 'milli-seconds'.

Double prefixes are not used. For example, since the base unit of mass – kilogram – already has a prefix, 1/1000th of a kilogram is not called a 'milli-kilogram' but a 'gram'.